MOTHER

I0223746

BY
L.A.WESTFALL

'One million people commit suicide every year'
The World Health Organization

All rights reserved, no part of this publication may be reproduced by any means, electronic, mechanical, or photocopying, documentary, film, or otherwise without prior permission of the publisher.

Published by:
Chipmunkapublishing
PO Box 6872
Brentwood
Essex
CM13 1ZT
United Kingdom

http://www.chipmunkapublishing.com

Proofread by: Jessica Houng

Copyright © 2007 L A Westfall

I dedicate this book
To Pam and Les Phillips
From Mersea Island
The best foster parents any child could wish for.

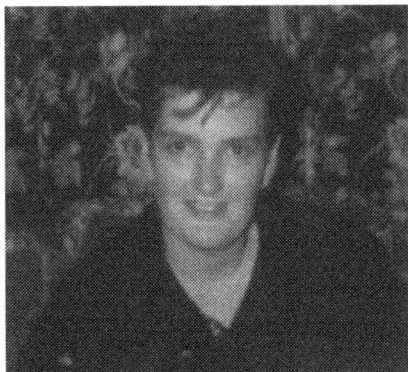

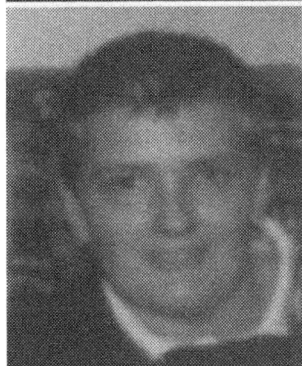

Prologue

My life began on September 8th the year 1962, the day the whole world of peace, loving and happiness died. Well for me it did anyway. My mother named me Lindsay, after someone she knew had died, hoping the same fate would befall me. She looked into my eyes and all I saw was evil and hatred.
I know babies can't see at a day old, but if I could that is what I would have seen.   For the eleven years I had to remain with her I never saw any different.

Mary, my mother, was separated from our daddy. All we ever heard from our mother was that he was a drunk and a gambler. I was too little to know if this fact was true or not.

I and my brother Arthur, who was eighteen months my elder, and our mother, lived together in a large house. It was easy to pick out; it was the one with the black sky over it, with no light in sight. Mother had to work part time because she had two brats to feed, and to go on any sort of welfare was too degrading. She got work typing in an office, Arthur and I went to Nan's and Granddad's every time she went. I think that's how we survived our early days, for we were very young and too easy to kill.

Mother was very mad but at the same time very clever.   Within a short space of time, she was all over her boss. A fat grey haired old man. I don't

know how long it took her to get him down the aisle, but that's just what she did. He was past his prime and just wanted to get a woman. But oh my God how he would regret it. He never saw the black sky until it was too late. My book is about my life and how it started, as I remember it; I aged five and Arthur aged six and a half years old or roundabout. In a large house with posh things, and pound signs everywhere; well he was the boss.

Chapter One

"I'm sorry, please, please mummy I won't do it again." "You stupid brat you evil little cow. How many times have I told you to go outside and brush that bloody mop of yours, how many times aye", and with that a hand with a rolling pin in it came down across my back. I fell to the floor. Again she rained her anger on me. I lay on the kitchen floor, feeling the coolness of the lino on my face, not wanting to move, not able to move.

"Get up you little bitch, I haven't finished with you yet." Suddenly she grabbed my hair from the back and yanked me to my feet. I closed my eyes because even at a young age I knew there was far more to come. There is no fury like our mothers. "You won't do it again." With that she grabbed my arm and pulled me into the dining room. "Get that chair you good for nothing little brat", she said. I obeyed as I always did; I put the chair on the path in our back garden and awaited my fate.

"Sit down and don't dare move". I was shivering, my back and rump were alive with pain, and I put my hand on my back and felt it lumpy. She came out of the back door with such fury I felt the house shake, I thought about Arthur. I knew he would be shut away in his bedroom; she always did that. No

eyes can even see that of another helpless child. With force that only evil had, my mother grabbed great chunks of my medium length brown hair, and started to hack at it, snip, snip the pain rained through my small body with such force, I felt I must die. Mother had pulled my hair so hard; chunks had been pulled out by the roots. At last her task was done and she went indoors calm and fulfilled. I remained on the chair frozen to the seat. My whole body ached with pain, can I move or should I stay. It seemed like hours but I suppose it wasn't; calmly my mother came outside with a dustpan and brush and told me to clean it all up, then come inside. I sat with the brush and pan and hoped that my body would allow me to do as I had been told. I emptied the dustpan of hair into the dustbin outside and returned the chair to the dining room from where it came. I returned to the chair I was sitting in, in the front room. Mother kept looking at the clock on the wall. I knew what she was waiting for; the return of the money man; Arthur and my stepfather William. We did not fear him; he was as scared of mother as we were.

Mother returned to the kitchen and started to prepare dinner. I remained in my safe chair. Arthur remained shut away. Time was soon approaching, my body was on fire, and my head had blood on it, when I touched it, but it was not long before William would be home and we would be safe.

Mother went upstairs and returned with Arthur; he was told to lay the table. My brother kept looking across at me with tears in his eyes. God knows what I must have looked like. We were summoned to sit at the table like we were every night, and await our stepfather's arrival. The key went in the door, no noise he made, for he was like us, he had to do as he was told. We heard footsteps on the stairs, as he had to remove his suit and office clothes the minute he came home.

Mother was putting food on the plates and winding herself up again, oh no God no more. We heard William coming down the stairs and opening the door; "Hello Mary; good day?" He looked at my brother and me then he gasped "What's happened to her". "Don't ask just don't ask" mother yelled. "I turned my back for five minutes and she starts cutting off all her hair". I tell you, I just don't know what to do with the little brat anymore. She needs a firm hand you know. William I am at the end of my tether with that little bitch. I wish I never had her." And then mother covered her face.

"There, there darling I know no one can do a better job of bringing up the children than you can, we will sort it out". There was no point in saying anything or looking funny, I had tried it all before. Arthur and I kept our eyes down and our mouths shut. Why cant he see my bald patches, the blood on my head, I ask you how could a five year old have done that to them self. But William like

everyone else only saw what they wanted to see. Our mother was a very clever woman.

Even at such a young age I knew what hatred was because every bit of my body and soul hated her. Why were we made? I thought about this for a long time and always had the same answer. We were toys for mother to do with what she liked.

Chapter Two

Arthur and I went through the rituals as we did every morning for getting ready for school. Our beds had to be made just the way mother liked them, our night clothes folded the proper way. Our teeth and face washed; our hair - well not that I had much left - combed out in the garden; even to eat was not a pleasure, the spoon had to go down on the table between each mouthful, and eat with your mouths closed at all times. I think that's why Arthur and I were so very thin, we never enjoyed food. Plates washed and put on the rack the correct way. Coats and shoes put on outside the front door, come rain or shine. Our lives were governed in every way, even down to going to the toilet.

Walking to school was very nerve racking, Arthur and I two steps behind silently carrying our school bags, never looking anywhere but in front, just like ants following the queen. Mother would reach the school gates and even without looking at us, she would do a quick about turn and head off to her perfect home. (Well it was until three o'clock when the brats return).

School life for Arthur and me was bliss, no pain, no fear, and no evil. No one ever hurt us; we did not know those teachers couldn't beat us. Sometimes teachers would ask me how I had hurt myself. I always had a ready prepared answer from mother for them, and I always obeyed. Arthur

was not as strong as me, maybe because he was never beaten, but the mental torture was just as bad for him. I know he felt guilty sometimes that the beatings I got, were for something or nothing that he had done. I never blamed my brother for anything; it was he and I against the whole world. As times went on our lives stayed very much the same. Arthur moved up to junior school, he was eight now, and he was getting a lot taller than I was, I remained in the infants.

I think it was about this time I began to realise that maybe every mother was not like ours. For William was, I think, just as scared of mother as we were but in an adult way. He was given some rules of the happy home that I am sure he did not like. Mary was his wife and his God told him, to love, honour and obey till death do part, so he let mother rule with an iron fist. I at this age felt sorry for him although Arthur and I never liked him one bit. He was weak and a coward, but we were not his children and to him that meant a lot, blood and all that.

If anything, mother was getting more evil, if that could be at all possible. There seemed to be times when she was meaner than others, not that you could enjoy the other times.

Nightmares were becoming worse; I went to my bed at night and shivered. I shall explain mother's new game, in the black of the night when the house was asleep, mother would creep into my

bedroom and suddenly I would awake in a choking tremor, for my mouth was covered by her hand. I would gasp fighting for my breath, eyes white with panic, she would warn me not to make a sound, then pull me from my bed and take me into the hall. There I was placed against the wall and firmly told not to move. I did as I was told, scared of what my fate was going to be. Suddenly I noticed that in her hand she had a rolling pin, oh God please help me. Mother said, "If you move an inch away from the wall then it's my turn to play", I didn't understand, is she going to beat me, or not. William's only in the next bedroom or is he? I didn't know.

Arthur's door was closed, I was so scared, I was shivering all over and I supposed I had moved, because suddenly down came the rolling pin, across the tops of my legs, I cried out with pain, and her hand was pushing across my mouth again. After what seemed hours she removed her hand, looked into my eyes and said, "Like my new game darling."

I stood for what seemed hours with my back, legs, and heels, touching the wall, my legs burning with pain. Mother was moving about the house upstairs, downstairs, in and out of rooms. William was not even in the house, I felt sure of that, when I could see a little light shinning in through the hall window. Just then mother shouted up the stairs and told me to get my arse in bed. I walked from the upstairs landing into my bedroom as if my

body was frozen. I tried to look at my legs but could not see very well. I could feel the intense pain she had inflicted upon me; she had done a good job this time.

Next morning still no William; he was always there when we first got up in the morning. My legs were mauve and red. I showed Arthur while we were still upstairs getting ready for school, but could not tell him about my nightmare of a night. I knew he could tell; sometimes it was only having Arthur that made life worth living.

We followed mother to school; I could not walk properly. Mother kept turning her head and giving us the evil eye. As we got to my school, instead of mother and Arthur keeping on walking, mother stopped and bent down to my eye level and said, "You rode your bike into a lamp post". With that she kept on marching. I looked on for a minute and saw Arthur wave from behind his back.

School was not so good now. Arthur wasn't with me. I missed him, I had no one else, no one, and I knew he felt the same. As always my explanation for my injuries was believed by all concerned. They had to believe what I told them or else mother would kill me. At times I prayed for that; but I had to think about my brother Arthur. Although he was older than I, he was not as strong as I was. I had to stay quiet for his sake, as well as mine. I had quite a brain for one so young. Next year I would be with Arthur. I could not wait:

play times, dinner times, it was the only time we had together, when we could be ourselves anyway.

As we fell into a march on our walk home, we knew something was wrong, but what? William it had to be, had gone away, had been killed, had she killed him? If William was dead or gone what about us? Arthur and I had no feelings for William at all, but we were safe when he was with us. We arrived at the house (for it was not a home) and we undressed from our school uniform. We were told to go into the play room and remain quiet, something is going to happen, (we were never allowed in there, it was only for show). We were right, a short time later William arrived home with someone; I think it was his mother. They entered the living room. Arthur and I played near the open door, to try to hear what was going on. Loud voices were coming from the living room. They were mother's. As Arthur and I tried to understand them; mother stormed into the dining room and kicked the play room door shut. Then she marched back like a soldier into the front room. Arthur was scared; he grabbed me and started to stutter trying to get his words out. He always talked like that but not with me, with me he could talk properly. When he was calm I put my arm around him and told him everything would be all right. I myself was praying in my head that William would not leave us. Raised voices and some shouting from both sides carried on for quite a while, we could not make out any words, but

mother was angry and that only meant one thing, I had to be on my guard.

The light in the garden started to fade and we had not yet eaten. We had not heard any voices for a long time. Arthur wanted to go to the bathroom for a wee wee. So did I; could we come out of the play room yet? We hadn't touched anything so mother couldn't tell us off for that. "Please Lindsay I need a wee come with me please," said Arthur, I don't know I said to him. We were told to stay here. Arthur needed the toilet so bad; so did I. Come on, I will go first. I opened the door of the playroom and crept through the dining room, we stopped at the door to the toilet. No voices, nothing, the coast was clear but where was mother. Arthur had a wee then I had one too, "don't flush the toilet" my brother said, she will hear, we went back to the dining room door but something was wrong, I felt a shiver run down my back.

I sent Arthur back to the playroom and told him to wait for me there. I returned to the hall past the toilet towards the front door, it was all silent. Were they asleep or just dead, had mother killed them both, I had to find out; I put my hand on the door handle and held my breath. I slowly pushed the handle down and clicked it open. I pushed it ajar still holding my breath, and put my head in around the door "I sighed thank God" the rooms were empty but where were they? The room was the same as I remembered it from this morning,

nothing broken, and nothing out of place. They must be upstairs, I started to creep upstairs one step at a time, my head was spinning I was so scared. I reached the top. All the doors were open. I checked the bathroom, it was empty. I also checked my room; it also was empty. I went across to Arthur's room; that was also empty. I built up enough courage to put my head into mother's room; that was empty as well. It was all very strange, so I went and looked out of the window. William's car was not in the drive. Both gates were open "we are alone Arthur" I shouted down to him. It is ok, come upstairs; I went back into mother's room. Arthur came running up, "Lindsay where are they?" said Arthur. "I don't know", I replied, "but Williams's car is not here, it has gone". "Gone, yes, we can get some food now, I am starving", said Arthur. "I don't know; they might come back anytime. I think we should go back to the playroom and just wait". "Please sis please I'm starving" said Arthur. "Ok but we will have to be very careful".

We went back downstairs, I knew it was wrong. We were not to touch any food (food was only pure if mother did it - only she knows how clean it is). I opened the fridge and took a packet of ham out, got the margarine and put them on the worktop. There were twelve slices of bread; she would not notice two gone. I took them from the middle and replaced the loaf as I had found it. Arthur and I made a stand in the front room so we could keep an eye out for them returning in the

car. I made the sandwich for Arthur and put everything back the way it was. I cleaned away the bread crumbs, wiped down the work surface and washed the knife and put it away the way it was. I had to keep Arthur's sandwich in my pocket so as not to get any crumbs on the floor. I checked everything again to make sure. Arthur was still keeping guard at the window. I called him and then gave him his sandwich, telling him to eat it quickly in case they came back.

We sat in the dark, just talking about what had gone on; we were both worried about William and the old lady. It was only nine forty five; we were six and a half and an eight year old and had been on our own for about five hours. I was angry because if we had known we could have played with some of the toys, and returned them back the same way. I looked at Arthur; he was very tired so was I; at least tonight I could sleep without fear. We both went to the toilet and started to go upstairs, I don't know what made me look at the front door, I suppose I just did. I reached for the handle and tried it; it was locked. Why; why was it locked? Mother had locked us in so no one could harm us, or so we could not get out? I went to bed with that thought in my head. Suddenly I was awoken by a fear that I had not had before. My eyes took a while to make out who was there, standing at the side of my bed. "Wakey, wakey darling mummy is back". A terror ran down my back for I had seen her like this before. Did you miss your mummy did you? I duly replied "yes". "But you managed to

disobey me didn't you. I told you to stay in the playroom didn't I." "Sorry mother, we were cold and needed the toilet, we did not know how long you would be." "Excuses, excuses; I was only gone for ten minutes. You will pay for disobeying me my girl". With that mother was gone. It would be about six months later that we were to find out what that night was all about, and how it would change our lives

Chapter Three

As Arthur and I both went to the junior school now, mother let us walk to school together. She would stand outside our house and watch us until we went around the corner of our street and out of sight. We could then run, jump, laugh, talk and be free.

School was the same play times, dinner times. Arthur and I could be together. We both enjoyed school; it was our escape from the nightmare we were living in. We both had a few friends of our own but we liked being together the best. After school we would meet at the gates as always. As we walked home our moods grew silent and fearful, and as we went round the corner into our street we walked like robots. I was thinking about something Arthur had said; he said mothers getting fat. Was she? I didn't know, I never looked at her (just through her). Tonight I would see.

As always the front door was on a jar; we removed our shoes and coats, bags and stepped into the hall. We both put our shoes on the stand and our coats on the peg and went through the hall with our bags to the dining room and kitchen. We took our places at the table and took out our homework from our bags, (even if we did not have any we still did some; we were safe until our homework was finished). For about ten to fifteen minutes we were writing when we heard the front door go. "Watch out, mother's about". She entered the

kitchen, like an actress comes on stage; our eyes remained on the words we were not reading.

Mother was getting food ready for dinner and never a word spoken unless from mother. Arthur's question kept going around in my head, was she getting fat, I didn't remove my eyes from my page, because you never knew when she was looking at us. Arthur gave the signal; a tap under the table. It meant that he had done his homework. I had also finished so in unison we started to pack our schoolbooks away. As we put our chairs under the table I glanced a look at mother but she had her back to me. Our school bags hung in the hall; we went to sit in the front room. We had a large television, but we hardly ever got to watch it because mother had the music on a lot. Arthur's place was in an armchair; mine was at one end of the settee - together but at arms length.

Bang, argh, mother was hurt. Arthur and I ran into the kitchen. Mother was on her hands and knees, she had dropped a saucepan. She turned a little and she saw us, she out-stretched her arm and grabbed mine. "Come here you little bitch look what you have done now, you will pay for this". Mother threw a cloth at me and told me to get this mess cleaned up. As she passed, she gave me a slight kick in my leg.

Mother grabbed Arthur's arm and dragged him up stairs. He was crying and mother was shouting at him. I heard him being put in his room and that

only meant one thing, I was in for it again. Mother came back downstairs and closed the hall door behind her. She entered the kitchen very slowly with her hand behind her back. I froze; please mother, please no. Mother's hand came upon me with fury time and time again, the wooden shoe thrashed me on my legs, bum, back and head, I screamed with pure pain and agony that only made matters worse. I lay on the kitchen floor unable to move, mother kicked me again "get up you little brat get up". I knew I had to, but I was unable to move. I was falling in and out of consciousness; then nothing.

I awoke the following afternoon in my bed, in my nighty. I moved my arms to move the bed clothes. As I did this I saw my arms. They were black, red, green and purple, my legs were the same. I pulled back my nighty and my belly and chest had quite a lot on, but not as much as my arms and legs and my head really hurt; even my eyes were sore. God why did I have to wake up; why couldn't this have been it? Then I thought about the only thing I ever loved; Arthur. That's why I had not died last night. I need to keep him safe. I went into the bathroom and went to the toilet; I looked in the mirror, I turned and turned back; amazingly my face was not hurt thank God for that I said to my self. I returned to my bed and slept again.

A hand was nudging me, "Lindsay, Lindsay are you all right, I thought you were dead, I was sure you were dead. I cried all the way to school.

Mother, she is evil I hate her. I will always hate her until the day I die." "Don't say that, don't ever say that", I told Arthur. "Keep your mouth closed and you will make it" "But what about you? We will see big brave brother, for you will live for both of us. "Don't say that Lindsay we will fight together." "Arthur, go to your bedroom before she catches you in here". Arthur kissed me and left; I had tears in my eyes, and I hurt so much.

Arthur always made me cry. He was older than me but much weaker. I was always the one to get the beatings, never him. I don't know why but I never took it out on him, for he could not have taken a beating not even one I felt sure of that. William came home; I heard them in the kitchen. Believe it or not I was hungry; it had been two days since I had eaten any food.

I waited to be told to come down for some food or some food to be brought up to me, but no, no food for the wicked, for I must have been very wicked.

Arthur put his head around my door and blew a kiss and was gone. I lay awake for a very long time because my tummy was making funny noises; I was so hungry. No one came to check up on me, thank God, because I lay in my bed and I cried silently into my pillow - for being so bad and evil, to keep getting beatings, I must be better, I must be braver, this beating nearly took all the fight out of me, but thinking of Arthur and how he needed me, made me realise I had to go on.

I heard William leave for work, mother came to the bottom of the stairs and shouted for both of us to get up and get dressed. To this day I don't know how I managed to put my clothes on, my whole body was in agony but I did as I had been told.

Downstairs Arthur sat eating his cereals at the table. I took my seat and started to pour my cereals into my bowl, then the milk, we were never allowed sugar on anything. Mother put a letter on the table beside me. "Give that to your teacher, it just tells her how you fell downstairs right?" "Yes mother". I put it in my bag. We both went into the hall and put on our shoes and coats. I could not bend down to tie my shoe laces. Arthur tied them for me and did up the buttons on my coat. We walked in silence to the bend of our road then once round the bend all hell broke loose.

"I thought she had killed you, when you did not come down stairs yesterday for school, oh Lindsay I missed you so much. Kids at school asked where you were. I did not know what to say". I told him "Just stick to what mother said and we will be ok".

"Are you in real bad pain", Arthur asked, "No, it is a lot better this morning" I replied. I just could not tell him the truth; how I really felt.

I don't know how but my body seemed to get better. And mother, well she was in a world of her

own. One day she didn't even cook any dinner. William came home and went straight back out, he was only gone ten minutes; he had got fish and chips. She still never moved from her chair in the front room. I didn't think she was very well, she had been funny for a week or two (not that I minded).

We ate in silence; mother never touched hers. William asked mother if she had seen the doctor today. Mother said "Yes any day now". "Right", said William, "Tonight we will get ready, ready". Any day now, what was mother going on about, ill, into hospital, well maybe she will die, oh that would be a prayer answered. I looked across at Arthur and he was thinking so hard I could almost see his brain working.

Mother looked different. For one thing, she had her big floppy house coat on. She would only wear that for doing the house cleaning. I think her face was not the same; "weird"! I don't know what it was, but it was not right. For the next hour the TV was on and we all sat in our places in silence staring at the screen. But not mother her eyes were closed. Yes, yes she is going to die, please, please God let her die in pain; thank you I said to myself.

We were sent to bed and William asked us to be quiet because mother needs her peace and quiet at the moment. At the top of the hall Arthur and I talked softly for a while then went to our

bedrooms. I think we are going to get a good night sleep. Sleep well my children no harm will come to ye this fine night and we both did. Morning shone through my bedroom window; I had forgotten to draw the curtains.   I jumped out of bed with a spring in my feet and sparkles in my heart. Was this the day my prayers had been answered? Arthur was awake; I pleaded with him to get out of bed and come down stairs but he was too frightened. "Please Arthur please, come with me, you want to know if mother is dead, don't you". "No, no I don't want to know. You go, leave me alone", said Arthur. "What's wrong", I asked. He replied, nothing, nothing. I said yes there is come on Arthur.   "I am scared. If mother dies we will get another one and what if she kills you and me as well".   "Oh Arthur come on I will always look after you. You know that."

With reluctance Arthur took my hand and we walked down the stairs very slowly. We walked into the hall and up to the kitchen door, my hand raised to open it. The door opened and Arthur caught the door and held it. "I am scared Lindsay lets go back upstairs and wait for mother". "No come on and don't be a baby."

I opened the door and went in. William was asleep at the table with his head on his arms. We both looked on in amazement, for we had never seen a sight like this before. I crept to the front room and looked in; it was empty so I went back upstairs and looked into mother's bedroom. She was not

there. I returned back downstairs to find Arthur still in the hall. We both stood and looked at each other; suddenly I looked at the coat pegs and shoe rack. Mother's were not there. I stood and thought for a moment; do they take dead peoples coats and shoes to bury them in. I don't know but there is only one way to find out. So we entered the kitchen and started to get the cereal bowls and get the spoons out. Arthur poured the corn flakes and I got the milk. After I put the milk away and went to get the sugar, Arthur said "We are not allowed sugar you know that." I replied, "Who says so" and that's how I recall now the first time I had ever defied her and you know it felt good.

We sat at the table silently eating our breakfast with William still asleep. I felt a warm glow all over my body; we were free, no more beatings, no more standing up all night, my prayers had been answered. I said, "Thank you God".

We finished our breakfast and went outside to brush our hair. Every morning we stood in our back garden brushing our hair, but this morning it was very different; there was a bird singing and the sun was trying to shine. The world felt a happy place. All thanks to my prayers. I don't feel guilty; I don't feel sorry or even sad for our mother. She was a very evil person; everyone knew that: Nan, granddad, William, Arthur and I; but not one of them had the guts to stand up to her and do anything about it. Until now. God did it; I shall pray for his thanks every day of my life, for I have

a life now, a future and maybe some happiness, and love; lots of love. I don't really know what that is but I know it is good.

With our hair brushed we went back inside. William was not in the kitchen, his chair had not been put back under the table. Mother would have cursed him for that. We both stood in the kitchen waiting for William to return. Arthur was shaking, I wasn't in my glory. William came in the kitchen and started to make a cup of tea. He didn't even look at us. I felt brave, I felt strong for the first time in my whole life. "Father where is mother?" I asked, he replied, "She is in hospital, so after school we shall go and see her, now off to school and don't be late", "Is she going to die", Arthur asked. William replied "Don't be stupid boy she has had a baby". I said, "She's had a baby". "Are you two bloody stupid or something, you must have known your mum was pregnant." We stood there and just looked at him. "I thought mum was dead." "Why would you think that", he replied, "Childbirth is Gods way; you have a beautiful baby she is your half sister; we named her Mandy. Now get a move on and get to school, hurry home tonight we will go straight to the hospital."

One minute ago my whole world looked happy and peaceful and all of a sudden it had all gone. Mother's alive, and to make it worse I now have another to protect. We were both silent on our way to school. I felt worse than I ever had before. I am only seven and a half and now I have two

children to protect, but in my heart somewhere I know I must for I can deal with dying but they can not. I had to explain what step meant to Arthur how she is not our real sister because William was not our real father. For the age of my brother he was not very clever.

All day at school I felt it was a dream God could not be so mean. At school they had taught us that God was good. All of it was a lie; I shall not believe him again. I felt totally lost; I waited for Arthur at the gate; we walked home to await our fate. William was dressed in his office clothes, clean and very happy. "Put your bags away and we will go; I bet you both can't wait", said William. "My daughter is beautiful. Your mother and I are very happy. We are a family now." Were we not before I asked myself, no I suppose not.

The ride to the hospital was silent. Arthur was the first to speak. "Where will the baby live?", he asked. "Well with us of course, where do you think she will stay", William replied. I answered for Arthur, "I think my brother means how long till she comes out of hospital." "I don't know; a few days probably. We have to get all the baby things set up for her. Mandy will sleep in our room for now but when she gets older you will share a room with her Lindsay. I know you won't mind, oh I can't wait until you see my beautiful baby".

Ward thirteen - that's a laugh for a start. Second bed on the right; mother was asleep she looked

peaceful, maybe the evil has gone now she has had a baby.

William went round the bed to a crib that stood on a stand; his eyes shined like I had never seen before. For a minute I felt happy for him but for only a minute. William waved for us to join him. We three of us all stood around the crib looking at this baby, and she had a pink jumper, and a hat and even a pink blanket on her. Looks are deceiving; mother suddenly woke up with a jump. As she opened her eyes she looked at us. I knew nothing had changed; God help us all. Mother was weak but she was still the same person; the first words to us were not I miss you both or this is your new sister they were "Why didn't you change your uniforms".

Over the next week mother and Mandy came home. A big hard pram, a high chair, a play pen and lots of clothes, toys and bottles appeared from nowhere and life carried on much the same as usual. Babies cry a lot, well in this house they do.

Chapter four

Well I don't know how I made it but I have just turned nine years of age, and my brother is now ten and a half and little Mandy; she is walking. William is very happy, he is always picking little Mandy up, mother shouts at him to put her down, you will have a spoilt little bitch if you don't leave her alone. Of course William obeyed; he always gives in, he never argues with her. He is what I think you would call a coward. Arthur and I feel sorry for him; he is a victim too.

It was just another day as Arthur and I walked home from school. If only I had known what lay in store for me on my return home from school. I think I would rather have jumped in front of a bus.

The front door was ajar; as always we hung up our coats, put our shoes on the rack and went through the hall to the kitchen to do our much loved home work. Mother was at the sink. I felt something was wrong. She turned to face us with such fury. In her hand there was a knife. Arthur cried out, I stood frozen to the spot. "Get to your room now", mother bellowed at Arthur. He turned, dropped his bag and ran. I gazed into her eyes and knew my fate. This was it, the day of my death by a knife; I didn't think, when this day would come, I would feel afraid, but how wrong I was.

Mother started yelling at me, "You horrible little bitch. I spend all my life cleaning up your crap

and are you grateful, No and that little bitch has been screaming all day, you, you're the worst. Now you will pay. Mother started walking towards me the knife firmly in her hand. I was trapped, I ran to the first chair by the table. She kept coming. So I pulled the chair out and kept going around the table. Mother was still screaming at me, "Bitch Bloody Bitch; wait till I get my hands on you". I had gone around all the chairs; still she came. I ran through the hall jumping over my bag as I went, I started to run up the stairs when I heard a big bang, and mother yelled out.

"You will pay for this Bitch". My God she fell over my bloody bag. At the top of the stairs I was trapped; where can I hide. I ran into mother's bedroom, I opened the white sliding door and got in. I pulled the clothes down to cover my head and face. She was upstairs I could hear her throwing things around, shouting her head off. I was frozen; I could not move. Suddenly I realised I was wetting myself. Within thirty seconds the sliding door was slammed open. "You bitch my clothes you little bitch", the knife still in mother's hand. She grabbed my hair and yanked me out of the wardrobe and she pushed me down onto her bed just below the pillows. Suddenly she screamed out and the knife came down to kill me. Just at that point mother stabbed the knife right into the pillow beside me.
Still with my head down she grabbed a bottle of spray (hair spray I think) and started hitting and

screaming at me, blow after blow she rained down on me, then nothing.

I know now as an adult I must have passed out. For when I awoke I was in bed naked. My face felt like a balloon, my eyes would not open, my lips were fat. I tried to move but I just cried out in pain. In the days to follow I saw my body a mass of bruises that you would never think possible. Why had mother not killed me? Oh why? I cried a lot in the week I remained in my bed unable to move. Arthur was ordered to bring my food up. He was so scared without me. I felt for him and little Mandy but I was just too weak to help them.

Mother didn't let me go back to school for quite a while - about two weeks or so; until my bruises had faded. I had the flu, it said in her letter and I was told to say the same. (Didn't teachers think I was ill a hell of a lot)? Mother never went to our school, never. William went to the parent evenings, plays, sports days, etc. etc. The loving step father in a lot of ways, he was just as bad as mother, because he pretended nothing was happening, he always looked the other way, MOTHER RULED O.K.

Mother was very clever. She always had an answer but not this time. Sally's mum from the end of our road knocked on our door one day after school. Mother was very angry when she had to get up and answer the door. "Hello Mary you know I was telling you about Sally's new brownies club.

Well I told them about you and your Lindsay and how reputable you are. And they said they would welcome Lindsay into the group, I just had to come and tell you straight away, I knew how happy you would be".   "Oh right, yes right", mother said, "I will have to think it over".   "But Mary, they only have one place she will have to start tonight or lose the place. I tell you what I will do I will drive her there and bring her back home with us, it's such a pleasure to help such a nice family like yours. I will pick her up at six o'clock on the dot, bye, bye for now see you later".

Mother shut the door and came back into the front room, gob smacked; one nil to Sally's mum. Brownies, well I don't really want to go but it will get me out of the house once a week; but would mother allow the lady from the end of our road to win. Mother sat for a long time deep in thought. I dare not move an inch. Mandy was asleep in her playpen, Arthur was in his bedroom drawing, (Nan had bought him some drawing pencils and a book and told him to do some pictures, mother had no choice she had to let him use them).

Mother lost. I don't know why she gave in, but I do know that Sally's mum had a big mouth. Six o'clock came and I was on the doorstep waiting. Brownies was quite good fun; we played games, made pictures; I had a very good time. But I couldn't get it out of my head; would I pay for it when I got home. I thought maybe not because William would be home.

When I arrived home the front door was ajar. I went in, hung my coat up, shoes went on the rack and went into the front room. William was in his chair in the corner. Mother was watching TV. Arthur was in bed I suppose and Mandy also. Without moving her head mother said to me "BED". I turned and obeyed straight away, I was safe, well for now anyway.

Life carried on much the same. Mandy was allowed out of her playpen sometimes, but life was not good for her; William was the only adult to kiss her or cuddle her, well Nan also.

We visited Nan and Granddad about every two months or so; she only lived in London. But it was hard for mother. Nan's flat was a warm and friendly home, ours was a SHOW piece. I don't think mother felt clean visiting Nan's. Mother always gave Arthur and me the same talking to every time we visited, don't say this or don't say that. Sit with your legs together, wipe the toilet seat before you use it and so on, these were the rules of visiting.

Nan and Granddad loved us I think. Granddad loved mother very much, I was always aware of that. So I don't think I allowed myself to get close to him, (as an adult I know that's a shame but as a child I didn't think he could have loved mother and me as well). Nan, well Nan was just great; she gave us cuddles and kisses and loving looks, oh if

only Nan was our mum. I remember on one visit, Nan was doing her washing in the kitchen; Nan had her mangle and her scrubbing rack and was hard at it when we arrived. It made mother feel sick, - old peoples washing. Nan said Arthur and I could help her. We were over the moon, mother was fuming and we knew it. But the pull was too strong, Nan it was. Arthur put the clothes in and I turned the handle. Nan pulled them out the other end. Arthur wanted to do the handle, Nan said, "All change". Nan put the washing in, Arthur turned the handle and I pulled the washing out. Suddenly Nan gasped, she grabbed my arm and pulled me up to standing position again. She lifted my jumper from the back and gasped again.

"What the hell happened to you child"? I couldn't look Nan in the eyes. She looked at my chest and ran her fingers gently over me so as not to hurt me. "What has happened to you child, tell Nan". I lifted my eyes up to see my darling Nan's face, "I fell", I said. "I fell over at school". At that moment mother came charging in. She had heard. She didn't look very happy. Nan sent Arthur and me into the front room with Granddad, William and Mandy. I crossed my fingers, toes and everything so that she would not hurt my darling Nan. I was afraid for her; she was very old - well to me as a child everyone passed thirty was old. We could hear raised voices in the kitchen. Granddad got up and quickly went into the kitchen to see what was going on. Even William was concerned.

After a few minutes the voices stopped, mother came out into the front room picked the little brat up and announced that we were leaving. William looked at mother as if to say what the hell now. But thought better of it and hustled us all out of the flat door. The ride home was silent. We were sent to our rooms for the rest of the day. Nothing was said; we didn't even get our dinner. We didn't see Nan and Granddad for a long time after that day. Nan never said anything to me but her eyes said it all, she knew.

Mother started a job. I don't really know what job; it was two evenings a week. I know it wasn't because she needed the money. "We are rich", she told us often enough, she bought her own car, a little red one. William was never allowed to drive it. "It was mothers". I don't know why the job, the car, but she seemed quieter so we were glad. She could have a fleet of cars if she wanted. Mother worked Mondays and Tuesday nights straight after our dinner. She seemed to enjoy it. Mondays I went to brownies but Tuesday nights were nice without her. William let us watch TV and he always played with Mandy. It was his time with his beloved daughter.

I would look at him and Mandy and would feel jealous. He loved her, she was lucky; at least she had one parent. Mother as far as I knew or saw never beat Mandy for fear of losing her meal ticket but was nasty to her in other ways. Mandy spent most of her first two years in the playpen in the front room; mother put the wooden highchair in the

playpen then Mandy in the highchair. Babies are filthy little brats - mother's words - so keep them "confined".   Of course if anyone came to the house Mandy was out of the playpen and the apple of her eye.

Mandy had a bed the same as mine in my room, now the cot was gone. Mother didn't do the night rounds so much now for fear of waking Mandy.

For as many fingers I have on my hand, I spent hours standing, back and legs straight against the hall wall, hour upon hour - it's funny, but out of all the things she did to me as a child, that was one of the hardest.

It was a normal day.   Arthur and I had arrived home from school, we were seated at the dining room table in silence when Arthur passed me a piece of paper - it was ok because mother was in the front room.   It said where do we live?   I whispered to him, "Here of course". He replied, "I need to write our full address and post code. I don't know it".   I looked at his face; he was scared.   The house number is eight, the name of the road is Fairhaven, I told him. "How do you spell that", he said.   I told him how I thought it was spelt. We had walked past the sign a million times on our way to school, I felt angry at him, he was the eldest. He should have known. Arthur sat and stared at me; if I don't get it right I will be held back, and then mother W-W-W-I-LL get mad.

"I'm sorry Lindsay, I know I should know but I don't, pl-e-a-s-e don't get mad at me". One look at my brothers eyes and I felt guilty, "Sorry", I said. I was wrong, "let me think a minute". I sat with my head in my hands trying to think of a way around it. "We will have to ask her; I don't see any other way". "B-B-U-B-U-T M-M-O-T-H-E-R W-W-I-LL G-G-E-T A-N-G A-N-G-R-Y". "Its alright Arthur. I will tell mother it's <u>my</u> homework then I will get told off, not you". "N-NO S-I-S-I-S that's not fair". I thought to myself, what's one more beating, but of course I didn't say that to Arthur. He was scared enough without making it any worse.

I took a clean piece of paper and like a tin soldier marched into the front room and stood near mother and waited to be spoken to. "Yes what do you want now? Can't anyone get any peace around here"? The fact Arthur and I had not laid eyes on mother since we left the house for school that morning left me a bit bemused.

"Sorry mother, but could you please write our full address and post code down for me, I need it for my homework". She looked at my outstretched hand with the paper and pen in it and I swear I saw her eyes turn red and then back to brown. "You're nine years old and you don't even know your own bloody address. You're bloody useless, you thick little bitch".
She grabbed the paper and pen from my tiny little hand and with fury wrote on the paper. I trembled on the spot too scared to move an inch. With

anger pouring from her body she stood up and grabbed me by the hair. And dragged me through to the kitchen. She threw me into the chair and slammed the paper in front of me. "Write it over and over again until I tell you to stop. I'll teach you, if it's the last thing I do you stupid cow". With that she went back through to the front room. Arthur came to me and cuddled me, "S-S-S-O-R-R-Y L-L-I-N-D-S-A-Y". "It's ok Arthur. It's alright, honestly I didn't get hit, now write it down quickly write it down in case she comes back in". Arthur quickly wrote the address down, then he returned it back to me. For the next hour I wrote and wrote and wrote 8 Fairhaven Road, Littleton, Essex, CO5 7PR.

I filled in the page front and back and sat waiting for mother to return. Arthur had done his homework and I told him to get upstairs out of the way. I sat thinking to myself that was too easy; when mother came in she asked why I was not writing. "I have done it", I replied, and held up the paper for mother to see. She went to the drawer in the kitchen and took a stack of paper out. She through it down on the table just in front of me and said "Well do it again, fill these as well". For a slight second I looked into her eyes; anger, anger was what I saw. I must be the worst kid in the world to make my mother so mad; it's my entire fault, I am a little bitch, I must be.

Dinner came and went, I still remained at the table writing; it's my own fault this time, it's not mother's

fault it's mine. She is right; nine years old I should know my address and post code. I heard later in the evening William and mother talking loudly. I heard my name said. Then I heard someone going up the stairs. My hand was really hurting. I had a blister on my thumb. I was tired but I kept on writing.

A while later mother came into the kitchen and washed up some cups, she tidied up the kitchen and then locked the back door; she went back to the kitchen drawer and took out more paper. Mother picked up the sheets of addresses on the eleven pieces of paper that I had filled. Without really looking at them she ripped them up in half then in half again. "DO YOU KNOW IT YET" mother yelled at me. "Yes I replied". "Well I don't think so you stupid bitch", she yelled back at me. She threw the new clean paper on the table in front of me and said, "When you fill them up then you can go to bed and not before". With that she turned and went through the hall and up the stairs to bed. It was my fault, all of it, I sat looking at all the paper and I sobbed.
I worked all night; I filled every page front and back with our bloody address, my right hand was covered in blisters, I wrapped toilet paper around them but it was still agony.

The light was coming in through the kitchen and playroom window. It will soon be morning, two more pages to go. All through the night, I had sobbed quietly to myself, if this was my fault -

maybe all of it was maybe - I am the evil one and not mother. All these thoughts were going through my head all night long. I feel so messed up and knackered I could sleep for a week - well only if mother wasn't in the house. Done all done. I tidied the table up and went to the toilet and got rid of the tissue from my hand. I washed my face; my eyes were red and swollen. I felt a right mess; I was coming out of the toilet when I saw William going into the kitchen. He turned and saw me and looked so guilty, for he was the adult and should have stopped it. I followed him and watched as he got some cereals out and placed them on the table. No words were exchanged but looks said it all, he was just as scared of her as I was. I sat and ate my breakfast in bliss for mother was still asleep.

Arthur was going up to secondary school come September. I would miss so very much. I still had my best friend; well my only friend at Grange Way junior school but it was only Arthur I could talk to and he to me as well. We knew we could tell no one because if we did we were dead (I can't write and express how bloody petrified of mother we both were).

In three weeks it would be the summer holidays, it was hell for both of us but for everybody else they just couldn't wait and talked of nothing else. One person only one person I would miss was Mrs Hook; she was a dinner lady at our school. I have learnt that if I looked sad enough she would let me

hold her hand sometimes and if that came about it would make my day. It was the touch, the warmth I felt from an adult, there was nothing like it. I would miss her during the long six weeks that lay ahead of us for school was our only escape.

Chapter Five

This is our last week at school. We were dreading the next six, we were washing and drying up the dinner things; mother had just left for work. Mandy and William were in the front room playing. Arthur and I were talking about how we were going to manage, when William came into the kitchen. He told me to get my uniform on. It was ten to six. I rushed upstairs quickly and got changed. Although at first I didn't like brownies I did now, it was fun.

Sally and her mum picked me up outside our front door and drove us to brownies each week. Nothing different or unusual happened that evening until I arrived home. Then God was I in for it? William was at the front door waiting for me; he had never done that before. He greeted me with open arms; I managed to squeeze past him and into the hall. I took my coat and shoes off and put them where they went. I started to go upstairs, when William said, "Come into the front room for a minute. I want to talk to you". I obeyed, no reason not to, "Where's Arthur", I asked. "He's having an early night. Now come over here and sit with your old dad". I froze. All the years mother and he had been married neither he or mother had never said dad or daddy, nothing like it, it was always "Father".

I walked over to where he was sitting very gingerly. "Sit on daddy's lap", William said, "Next I need a big cuddle from my big girl", (big girl, big

"Look darling, daddy's a big man isn't he?" Then he took off his shirt. I stood frozen. I had never seen a man (or woman) naked before. This is sex; I thought it must be but…. My step father lay down on the front room floor with a big cushion under his head. He said, "Come darling lay with daddy". I got a cushion and lay beside him. He turned on his side at that point. And he started touching and kissing me. I tried to push him away but he held my hands firm. He put his hand between my legs and started moving his fingers, this feeling went straight through my body. What it was I don't know, but I didn't like it. He was whispering in my ear.

Hand between my legs, he was moving his bum up and down. After a while he stopped and he told me to sit beside him; I didn't want to, I was scared but he would tell mother if I didn't. "Give me your hands" he said. I did as I was told. He put both of my hands on his penis and he showed me ho to move them up and down. "Now keep doing that until I tell you to stop, do you hear me". "Yes", I replied. I was crying; I don't know how long I did it for - not long I suppose - when he suddenly shouted at me to go faster. I did as he asked, he was moaning and groaning then suddenly he let out a yell, and he laid on the floor, flat.

Stuff that smelt awful was all over my hands; I panicked. I jumped off him and ran to the settee picking up my uniform and ran upstairs. I ran into

the bathroom locked the door behind me. I threw all my clothes in the laundry basket then turned the taps on to fill the bath up. I then turned the taps of the basin on, I started scrubbing my hands with the small nail brush with such fury I could not feel the pain, I scrubbed non stop until the bath was full. I got in the bath and started to scrub the rest of my body clean. All the time I was sobbing to myself, I felt dirty, I felt used, it was wrong, I knew it was wrong.

I remained in the bath for a long time, and then suddenly I panicked. Mother, she would be home soon. I got out of the bath to dry myself. Oh God what have I done. My body was red and so sore, I had scrubbed myself raw. I patted myself dry, put my nighty on and took myself to bed.

Over and over in my mind it played what had happened. Each time it made me feel even sicker, my eyes stung because of all my tears. How I got to sleep that night I just don't know but when I awoke it was morning. Mother was down stairs; well I hope its mother and not him. I lay in my bed trying to work out a way of ending my life. With both of them at me, I couldn't take it anymore. Death has always been a way out but Arthur and Mandy had always stopped me. But now, after the night I have just gone through

We never had any money of our own. I knew mother had a book with money in it for us; birthday and Christmas money etc., but even if I could get

at it, they would not let me have any I was sure of that. But I needed money, "money for pills". Mother had some pills, but they were kept in the medicine cabinet; she would know if I went within twenty feet of them. Come on Lindsay think, but I just couldn't, I just laid in my bed and cried, I just wanted to die; please God let me die.   I can't take anymore. P.L.E.A.S.E.

Four more days of school.   I walked all the way to school in silence.   Arthur kept on and on at me asking what the matter was (as if he didn't know, I was thinking he must have heard my cries for help). Still I remained silent for I was angry at him; he was my big brother. My teacher asked me three times if I was all right, each time I just said I was tired. I was in a world of my own. Jump in front of a car, climb up onto the school roof and jump off, shop lift for pills from the chemist and take them home. Take mothers big knife and cut my throat open, drink toilet cleaner from the down stairs toilet.   My whole day I spent trying to think of ways of ending it all.   I had had these thoughts before but not so real.   I had made my mind up; death was my only way out.

Home time finally came; Arthur was at the gate waiting I saw him and he looked so sad. I walked straight passed him without looking at him; he caught up to me and pushed me against the school fence. "What the hell have I done he shouted at me" "as if you don't know" I replied, but I don't, honest please please Lindsay I don't know. I looked into his eyes and all I could see was pain.

"Went to bed early last night did we". Yes he replied, William made me I was tired, I think I went straight to sleep, WHY what happened, I just looked at him he could be telling the truth, please, please Lindsay tell me what's wrong did you get a beating from mother. Well now I know he is telling the truth. We walked very slowly holding hands and I told him what had happened the night before. He didn't say a word his face said it all he went white as a ghost, we were about three-quarters of the way home when I had finished telling him what had happened. He grabbed my arm with love and gentleness and cuddled me, I'm sorry Lindsay I was asleep. Could you not fight him back, no I told him and explained what William had said about making mother angry. He is a great fat hairy bastard Arthur said. Listen Lindsay we can beat him and as long as we stick together and work as a team, what do you think. I looked at Arthur and said your being very brave aren't you (The minute I said I was sorry) I am only trying to help. I'm not and your not scared of him has not like mother is he, well no I replied but he will tell mother if I don't do as he says. Look, listen trust me we can beat him. I promise, but Arthur mother works tonight we will be on our own with him he could do the same thing. Trust me sister, he will not, please for once in my life I can help you, I love you more than anything in the whole world your all I have. I can't stop mother nobody can, but he is different. We went round the corner and fell in line like soldiers and entered our beloved home which held our beloved family.

Mother put her coat on and left for work Arthur and I couldn't take our eyes off of William, I was scared but Arthur was so strong (I had never seen him like this before). We had done the dishes so we had no choice but to go in the front room with him. My whole body was stiff with fear, (what if Arthur couldn't stop him). I can't go through that again. We sat and pretended to watch TV but of course we were waiting for the time to pass for Arthur's big moment. At seven thirty six William turned to Arthur and told him to go to bed. I looked at my brother fear in my eyes. "Come on sis" Arthur said time for bed. I rose from my seat and started to walk out of the door, William looked at me and said, get your nighty on then come back down I want to talk to you. I looked at Arthur, William saw me, don't look at him, he's a useless piece of shit. Now do as you have been told or I shall tell your mother how bad you <u>both</u> have been.

We went through the hall and up the stairs on the landing I panicked, what am I going to do? Arthur please you said "you could help fix it" oh my god what can I do I was crying. I was marching up and down the hall, help, help me Arthur help. "LINDSAY" William shouted up from the bottom of the stairs "get down here now if you know what's good for you." I stood at the top of the stairs and looked at my brother, slowly I went down one step at a time crying as I was going, Arthur remained in the top hallway watching me, I walked into the

front room not crying but sobbing. "You can stop it right now young lady if you know what's good for you. And with that he slapped me right across the face. Well I'm telling you and you can tell Arthur, if you think your life is HELL now, wait and see what I can do to you both if I can make mothers life hell just imagine what yours will be like, get the idea? Well you better. Now get up there and tell your bastard of a brother then get down here and do your duty." I ran upstairs and through my sobbing I revealed to Arthur what William had said. Tears in his eyes, for he knew as I did, we were beaten. I returned back downstairs and like the night before performed my daughterly duty.

Arthur remained on the upstairs hall he also was sobbing his heart out, for he had failed me, (the fact that we were both children didn't enter our heads). In the bathroom Arthur had already run me a hot bath, he helped me scrub and all the time he was crying with me. Don't Lindsay you're making your self-bleed", "I have to get him off me", I scrubbed and scrubbed until I could not do it any more, I stepped out the bath and Arthur dried me with tenderness. Arthur dressed me in my nightclothes and took me to my bed, he stroked my wet hair but it made me flinch every time he stroked it so quickly he stopped. I think he stayed with me until I fell asleep, but I don't know because I was in a world of my own.

About a year or so earlier I found a place that I could feel safe, I think it was part of a dream

to start with but it soon became more than that. If I concentrated really hard I could let my mind go blank. I could only do this when mother was out or asleep. At first I could only see a young girl dressed in a pure white nighty, but as time went on I saw and learned much more.

Her name is Lindsay; yes I know two Lindsay's are a bit weird, not really for there is only one. We are one person, she is safe I keep her safe and when I am with her I remain safe. I can only go to her sometimes, when I have been beaten or sexually abused, only sometimes can I find her. If I am not hurting then as long as I can concentrate hard enough I have a better chance of getting to her. I suppose it's like having an imaginary friend. It gave me comfort especially at night knowing that I have a friend in the dark. No one knows about her it is our secret for if I told I would surely lose her.

We are half way through our school holidays nothing had changed. Oh well one thing, I have no hair again, do you know why, just because I left a few hairs in my brush when I brought it in from the garden. This time I was lucky mother cut it off not ripped it out, but I do miss it I look like a boy. Mother is angry because I have lost weight, a lot as well; she kept on telling me to pull my jeans up which I did. Then one day when I had them on she called me into the kitchen and told me to lift my top up. I obeyed very gingerly fearing what was in store for me. And all she did was pull the waistband of my jeans and remarked

how big they were. "She asked me if my other trousers were the same" I replied "yes" a look came over her face I had never seen before (I know now for a child to lose that much weight is very worrying but then I was no ordinary child).

About a week later as good mothers should be I got two pairs of jeans thrown at me after one of her shopping trips. Mother hated all children, but especially me, and yet we all had nice clothes. Never any toys, that's a lie really Christmas, birthdays we were given things but only on a few occasions we were allowed to play with them, they would be put in the play room all in neat piles and kept for show.

One day a lady and a man knocked on the door during the holiday from the children's society, they asked mother if she could donate any clothes or toys to help the needy. Well straightaway mother invited them in and made them comfortable in the front room. "Arthur" mothers shouted when he came in. She told him to go into the playroom and bring two piles of games out, while mother was waiting for Arthur to return she told them how she always helped all the children's societies, all those poor little mites with nothing, "I feel for them all" she said. Arthur returned with the first pile, mother told him to get some dustbin liners. The man's face; as he looked at the first pile, "but these are new" he told mother, she replied "my children are so lucky they have so much. Please give them to all those who are

without". Arthur returned with the second pile and the dustbin liners and with lots of thanks they left. "Two faced cow" I thought, "you know they were new, only because you never let us play with them."

Mandy never meant much to me and Arthur, after all she was only a half sister but since William has started hurting me I can't seem to look at her and not see him. I think Arthur feels the same way. Anyway we have a plan, for the next time our stepfather needs a bit of sex, we are going to make him pay for it.

As if enough wasn't happening, mother started getting very moody again, with it she got very angry, and we know who gets the worst of that ME. My duty every morning was to make mine and Mandy's beds and dust the chest of drawers and shelves all before school. On Friday morning on the last week of the holidays I had done the bedroom and went down stairs for breakfast. Mother was not down here something felt wrong I held my breath, fear took hold of me Arthur felt it as well, he looked at me with fear in his eyes, "where is mother?" I whispered across the table. I don't know I replied but I am scared Lindsay, be careful, at that moment mother burst into the kitchen slamming the door so hard it could have come off its hinges. "Lindsay you bitch you fucking bitch how dare you touch my things" she started screaming at me, go in my room destroy my stuff would you. Well you're going to pay for

this now get upstairs". Mother tried to grab my hair but because it was so very short. She could not get a grip on it. So she grabbed my upper arm and dragged me behind her up the stairs. I was telling her I had not been in her room but she was yelling so loud. I could not understand what she was saying. But I could hear Arthur screaming for her to leave me alone. Mother grabbed my head and pushed it down onto the chest of drawers, "LOOK, LOOK, what you have done, you fucking bitch, how dare you touch my stuff". "I didn't, I wouldn't, please mother!" I shouted through my tears I have not been in your room "Don't give me that" with this she whacked me straight across the face, I fell on the floor, (mother was very strong especially when she was angry). She pulled me up and whacked me again about the head. I fell onto her bed; repeatedly she hit me until all her anger had gone. She stormed out of the bedroom and down the stairs where I could hear her shouting again. "Arthur oh my god Arthur" I said, I crawled to the top of the stairs; my face bleeding the shouting was getting louder. Arthur, Arthur I cried, I crawled half way down the stairs and fell the rest of the way, at the bottom I pulled myself up by the hand rail, still mother was shouting. I staggered along the hall and into the kitchen. Arthur was behind the table and mother was in front of it shouting her head off, she saw me the minute I came through the door and started coming towards me, "aren't had enough aye, well we will see about that". She picked up the bread board and started bashing my upper body with it, I fell to the floor and rolled up

into a ball so as to protect my head again and again the board came down on my back, then suddenly nothing.

I awoke in my bed naked; I looked across at Mandy's bed she was asleep in it. I tried to move but the pain was too bad, tears rolled down my face, my body and (my mind) could not take anymore. (I think that this time in my childhood I felt the lowest). "ARTHUR" oh god where's Arthur. I knew mother could kill my brother very easily. Arthur, Arthur I kept whispering his name for I knew if he was all right he would come. Nothing I whispered and whispered but no Arthur.

I have to see if he is alright, I have too, I moved the covers from my chest and tried to sit up, I yelled out with pain, I couldn't move, but I have too, again I tried to move, again I cried out in pain. I lay in my bed, a broken child. I cried so much Mandy woke up. SHIT, no please, Mandy its all right go back to sleep, I pleaded with her but she kept on crying. Foot steps on the stairs its MOTHER. She entered our room and went straight to Mandy's bed "what's the matter with you" mother asked "Lindsay's crying" said Mandy pointing to my bed she woke me up. Did she now mother replied, well she won't anymore, now go back to sleep? Mother came over to my bed and said "what's the matter with you". Normally I would not have answered back but I had to know if Arthur was still alive, "is Arthur all right I asked?" "Of course he is, now shut up and go back to

sleep if you know what's good for you", with that she turned and marched out of our room and down the stairs. I was glad I had woken Mandy up, for at least I knew my brother was all right.

During the night I woke and needed to go to the toilet, bad really bad, I again tried to move to get out of bed and again, I fell back in agony. She's broken my back, I'm sure of that. I can't move, my face feels twice the size it should be. My mouth tastes of blood (I need a wee) I need to go to the toilet, oh god if I wet the bed she <u>will</u> kill me, good I thought and I lay there and wet my self. When I had done I felt a relief come over me, now she would kill me, I fell back to sleep a happy child for tomorrow <u>I shall die</u>.

Tomorrow didn't come, mother realised she had really hurt me badly, I stayed in bed for at least two weeks I didn't even start back at school when everybody else did. She even fetched all my food up on a tray and she left me alone for a long time afterwards.

Arthur started Meadow View Secondary School; he looked really grown up in his new uniform and blazer. He liked it but he got lost twice in his first week, he hated going to school and leaving me at home with her, but there was nothing he could do, he had real home work and lots of it. I didn't see much of him for that first week and William I never laid eyes on him the whole time I remained in bed. Two weeks in bed was very hard in its self but my imaginary friend

Lindsay helped me a lot, when we were together nothing could hurt me "together we were safe". The feeling of peace and calm was so over powering. Sometimes I had to leave her room, but she understood, because she knew everything.

At last I could return to school, my first day was very lonely for I missed Arthur very much. Mother's letter and warning was that "I had the flu". Can you believe it all that time away from school; for flu? Well the teachers did I was given extra home work for a few weeks to try and catch up. I didn't mind Arthur and me could talk about our day while we did it.

At the weekend mother told us to put our best clothes on that meant we were going out to Nan's I hope. Yes were going to Nan's and Granddads. Thank you god mother gave us the usual lecture on the way in the car. Don't say anything sit with your legs together, wipe the toilet seat before you use it, we knew the rules off by heart we didn't care we just wanted to see Nan and Granddad. As soon as Nan set eyes on me she gasped and put her hands over her mouth "what's wrong Nan" I asked she put her hands around my face and kissed my head "oh my poor child" she whispered to me softly "you look so thin" "sh sh" I answered. Mother will make us go, she nodded she knew what I meant.

We stayed only for about an hour, mother could take no more of old people's houses she

thought they were all dirty even her own parents. I loved my Nan very much I didn't understand why she never helped me, well no one ever did well that's adults I mean I had Arthur and my Lindsay, I loved both of them with all my heart.

Our lives carried on much the same for a while, I think the last beating really scared mother for a while anyway.

Our plan for William was about to start, Arthur and me had worked it all out Monday night would soon be upon us.

Coming home in Sally's mum's car I was sick. "Sorry, sorry" I kept on saying thinking I must get hit for this. But no she kept on saying "it's alright dear lets get you home and tucked up in bed", as the car pulled up outside our house father came to the front door, he must have sensed something was wrong. I got out of the car and Sally's mum said; "now you get your self tucked up in bed". "I will call and see you tomorrow and see how you are". "Thank you" I replied walking from her car to the front door with William watching me it was like walking up the steps to hell. I had to tell William about being sick and that Sally's mum was calling tomorrow straight away William said, "that will please your mother" he had a grin all over his face. "You bastard I thought" I took my coat and shoes off and put them away I was just putting my right foot on the bottom step of the stairs when William grabbed my arm, "where

do you think you are going young lady?" "To bed" I replied "I am sick," "sick my arse get your self in the front room" "B-B-U-T I feel sick" I whispered as I walked into the front room. William was right behind me "stand here" he ordered I stood right in front of his reclining armchair; William took off his trousers, underpants, and shirt and sat on his throne. Like many times before he slowly undressed me his hands touching my body all over. He lay back in his chair and told me to sit on him. One leg each side of his legs his privates were touching me, I stared at the wall behind his chair and tried to go to my Lindsay, in her pure room I would be safe but nothing happened I just couldn't do it. William made me wank him until he came then like always I grabbed my stuff and went upstairs. Arthur was in the bathroom. GET IN he said he had filled the bath ready for me. As I got in Arthur threw my clothes to the laundry basket and gave the nailbrush. "Are you ok sis" I heard you say that you were sick, I replied "yeh in Sally's mums car" (I never knew Sally's mums name) "did she hit you?" Arthur said. "No" I replied, "she was really nice told me to go straight to bed. There is a but though she is calling round tomorrow to see if I am o.k." "Oh god mother won't like that" I know I said in the bath I was frantically scrubbing my hands, Arthur was washing my back, "come on Lindsay" Arthur had said "we only have ten minutes", "OK OK" I replied "but I have to get it all off". Arthur said; "stand up I will do all your back" I did as he had asked and between us we got all of me clean. Arthur tidied up the bathroom while I put

my nightclothes on. "Right" said Arthur "now we put our plan into action."

"You stay here and keep guard. If William or mother comes into the hall cough right?" "Ok, be careful please", "I will don't worry". Arthur went into mothers and Williams's bedroom, oh my god I kept thinking to myself; hurry up Arthur, hurry up. "Got it, now listen I'll keep it as planned until we set off for school. See I told you we could do it. He'll pay, sis I promise" at that moment we heard a car door, quick get in bed, mothers back, we ran like little rabbits being chased into there den. For the first time ever it was one nil to us, I tell you it felt good. It had worked out just the way Arthur had planned it; each week he would pay more and more, nothing in life was free.

In the morning at the breakfast table, I would look across at Arthur and all of a sudden I burst out laughing I just could not help it. Thank god mother wasn't in the room, Arthur's face looked angry as he told me to be quiet, "I'm sorry" I said I just could not help it, we sat for the rest of our breakfast just looking at each other, but inside I think we were laughing. Mother came down just as we were washing our dishes, I was waiting for all the shouting and screaming but there was none, instead she gave me a letter and told me to put it through Sally's mum's letter box on my way to school. Mother didn't look very good today I thought her face was a little white, maybe that's

why I got a letter, anyway I didn't care I just couldn't wait until it was time for school.

At the corner of the bend I posted the letter and Arthur and I ran further round the bend and down the road. Arthur stopped and leaned against the lamppost. And took off his shoe and his sock to take out the pound note he had, "hold it" he said to me so I can put my sock and shoe back on, I looked down and stared at the folded pound note in the palm of my hand. "Give it back to me sis" Arthur said, I held my hand out for Arthur to take it, he opened it and held it up to the sun to see if it was a real one, "yes" it's a real one a whole pound note. Just think what we can buy. I was just about to open my mouth when. Arthur said, "Only kidding honest". We both carried on walking to the drain that was a bit further on, (Arthur and me only walked half way to school together because my school was straight up and Arthur's was left past the shops) but by walking half way together was better than walking alone. Arthur and I stood side by side in front of the drain we could see all the dirty water at the bottom of it. Arthur ripped the pound note in half, he then gave me one half and just working like robots together we both ripped our half's into tiny little bits. "That was great," I said "yeh" Arthur said, then together we dropped our pieces down the drain. That's where William will end up if our plan works out all right, aye sis, "yes" I replied make him pay.

It was a few weeks since our first pound note that trouble was to follow me to school. It was normal playtime, I was playing with two other girls we were skipping when all of a sudden, a kid shouted out "LOOK OUT" and that's all I remember, until I awoke up in hospital with the worst headache of my life. I was on a ward, in bed, my head was bandaged all up and I had a tube in my arm, my eyes were a bit fuzzy, "where am I?" I kept on saying "Arthur where are you?" "It's all right" said a voice from my other side, I turned my head and a nurse was standing there. You had an accident in the playground of your school and you were brought here by ambulance. I have telephoned your mum "No please don't phone she's..." "she what?" "She doesn't like hospitals". "Yes I know she is sending your father to get you." "Now just lay back and rest, you will see your mum soon". I laid back and tried to think what happened in the playground, but it was all a blank. I dosed on my bed thinking to myself, I don't want to have any time off school because of it, I didn't want to have to be on my own with mother again.

Late in the afternoon William arrived he was not very happy, he had to leave work early, he nodded at me and went to the nurse's station. He was talking for a long time then he sat in a chair next to a wheel chair and the nurse came straight to my bed just like a bee to a flower. She explained that I could go home but I had to stay in bed for two to four days, "oh god please no" I said

with my eyes closed "what did you say child" "oh nothing I just don't like having to stay in bed", "oh" the nurse said, by the look of her eyes and face she wanted to say a lot more, gently the nurse took the tube from my arm and helped me put my uniform on, she told me as far as she new a metal netball post had fallen on your head, "don't you remember anything?" she asked, I replied "no nothing".

It was time to go home, holding the nurses hand we walked up to where William was sitting "there you go sir one daughter returned. Now look after her and don't forget plenty of bed rest". The minute I walked through our front door I was shouted at to go bed, I did as I was told for that was one very angry mother, as I walked into my room Arthur whispered "sis are you alright?" all of your school was talking about you. They said you were dead, I was so frightened, and "I'm ok just a headache" see you tomorrow. I undressed and was very glad to get to bed, for I only realised how much my head really hurt. I laid in my bed listening to mother and William arguing bad, real bad, but I was too dazed to listen to what they was saying, I slept well that night.

Mother was not herself, she still didn't look right, I think she was ill, but I was glad I know that was mean, but it meant no more beatings for a while and that was like winning the jackpot. My head felt better after a few days, mother told me to take the stupid bandages off. I stood up in the bathroom

and started to unwind the dressings from my head, pieces of hair were coming away with them, and I starred into the mirror afraid of what I would find. They had shaved all the very front of my hair; I had a great big cut about two inches long and about one inch wide, no stitches, but a skin dressing all over it. No wonder my head hurt, I looked really bad with my head shaven in the front, but to tell you the truth I was so used to being hurt, it was just another injury. When mother saw me without the bandages "she laughed" you sick bitch I thought, "I'm your daughter".

Things went very quiet for a while; mother didn't go to work, so William could not have his fun (when I look back at this period of time it was the best for years). Lindsay and I spent hours together at night when mother sent us to bed. It was so peaceful, we never left Lindsay's room, we couldn't but there was no need to, when I looked at Lindsay I didn't see myself for she might look the same as me, but she wasn't. Lindsay was safe she never got hurt, no beatings, no sex nothing, I envied her sometimes. But I was just so happy to have her, (for now as an adult, I know without her I would not have survived). No one knew about Lindsay, not even Arthur knew she was my secret, "just mine".

My hair has got a bit longer, but no hair grows on my scar, it still shows a bit, but I don't care with mother keep hacking my hair off. I was used to it. Mother recovered and started to work

again, Arthur and me was ready for our plan to start again. I thought of William's hands all over my body again it made me feel sick. But there was no way out of it, any of it.

Monday night came and went, William didn't touch me. Thank god I prayed, that night in bed, at last my prayers have been heard, (ha just shows how children think). For the following week I was not so lucky, again he stripped me and made me perform his sex games, he was very rough with me and bruised my upper arms badly, but unlike the last time my brother was not helping me to scrub myself clean. That night I lay in my bed crying I couldn't find Lindsay, and my brother had not come in to see if I was alright, I laid and felt totally alone.

Chapter six

I never write about Christmas, Birthdays, Easter or times like that for we never really had them. Yes we had a few presents each, but most of them just got put in the playroom. Cards were never put on display; they were shoved in the kitchen drawer. We never had cause for celebrations. I remember one-year coming up to Christmas. William said at the dinner table one day. "Shall I get a tree for the front room this year? It would be nice to be a bit festive for once". Arthur and I held our breaths for it came out of the blue. Mother looked at him with daggers in her eyes and replied "oh, you're going to hoover the mess up three times a day are you?" With that William looked down at his plate and said "yes you're right dear like always" the rest of our food was eaten in a ghostly silence.

Friends at school made Arthur and I feel sad sometimes. They talked about what they got, family parties, and exciting birthday outings. But I suppose if you never had it you can't miss it (rubbish) take it from me you can. Mother took more from us than anyone could know, little things like at the age of eleven and twelve and a half, Arthur or myself had never rode a bike, we couldn't, we never had one for I was thirteen before I learnt to ride, and that was at the home. Life carried on the same, the time passed slowly, but William was still playing his little games with me but last week as normal I went into mother's

bed room to collect my pay and Williams pockets were EMPTY. Next morning on our way to school I was very angry. William must have known what I had been doing. We parted company and continued to school. I was deep in thought for the big school holidays were coming up. And it was my last few days at Grange Way Juniors. It would be nice to be with Arthur again but I was a bit scared. Meadow View was such a big place and the holidays were always the hardest times for us because we were with mother all the time.

Friday last day of school, lots of kids brought cards, chocolates, and flowers for their teachers to say "thank you and good bye". Of course I was empty-handed. Only one person would I miss. My lovely dinner lady Mrs Hook, over the years she had been so kind to me as dinner time approached I felt scared inside, my belly was jumping up and down side to side silly aye, she probably wouldn't have realised that I had left. The bell went and I didn't go in for my dinner. I walked straight around to the second play ground to find Mrs Hook, I wanted to say good bye without the other kids listening, she was there, just like always. I walked over to her and as I got near she opened her arms to me, I ran the last bit and cuddled her so tight I thought my arms would drop off and without even knowing it I was crying. She pulled me to her side and said "hey there's no need for that" "but I will miss you" I said through my tears. No you won't she said you will be too busy with all them handsome boys chasing you

about, you will not have time to miss me. Mrs Hook cheered me up and cuddled me in her arms again you're a funny little thing you know. I cried again when the bell went and I had to walk across the playground and leave my dear friend "forever". Later as I left Grange Way for the very last time I felt nothing, nothing at all.

I have four more weeks of brownies then I have to leave. I like going but it was the coming home I hated, for Monday night was sex night (did I only have four more sex nights) he had already told me he could never do without me; I think the only way he would stop was if mother stopped work.

The weekend was no different to any others except for one thing William went out and when he returned he had a great big long box he took it straight out into the back garden what ever was going on, mother was not pleased. He was outside all afternoon. For he was no handyman. At last just before teatime we were all summoned to the back garden by William. Mother laughed loud as well "it took you all afternoon to put a swing up" and don't think your carting mud in and out because your wrong, straight away William said "no its not for them brats" pointing to me and Arthur "its for Mandy". (Talk about being treated like a bit of shit) "Oh well we will see" and with that mother went back into the front room with a smile on her face.

We sat eating our dinner it was a Monday so soon mother would be leaving for work, I was thinking how many times could I do it, it makes me feel SICK. It doesn't seem to me as if Arthur cares so much about me getting hurt by William anymore. I think he has got so used to it happening each week that is just part of our normal week; I wish I could feel like that if anything it is getting worse.

At brownies I was thinking if there would be any money. At first it did feel good that he was paying for it like a prostitute, but I just ripped all the money up so I didn't gain anything (not that I wanted his money I just thought if he had to pay for it he would stop). If I had known at brownies what lie in fate for me at home, I would have jumped in front of the first bus.

The door was ajar I hung my coat up and put my shoes on the rack, I knew not to go upstairs so I walked through the hall to the front room. William was in his reclining chair I went up and stood before him, "hello my darling I didn't hear you come in" (you liar I thought). Tonight my darling I have something a bit special for you. (Oh my god what now I thought) William called me to stand in front of him. Just like always he undressed me, his hands were all over my body then he stood up and undressed himself, not just his trousers his pants, his shirt everything, he took my hands in his and gently pulled me down on the floor with him. I was scared what was he going to

do now he kept whispering that he loved me and couldn't live without me and all the time he was kissing my body all over. Then he put his hand between my legs and he was putting one of his fingers right inside me. He was still talking and then he started sucking one of my nipples it hurt, but I could not speak I was in like a trance this carried on for a short while then suddenly he laid right on top of me. I gasped I could hardly breath. "Now for my special surprise my darling". With that he thrashed his penis into me; I cried out in pain, he put his hand over my mouth and with each thrust of his body his penis was going further in. Tears were rolling down my cheeks I cried but no sound came out. He took his hand away and kept on up and down up and down he said. "See baby I told you that you would love it" after what seemed like ever he roiled off me and lay beside me on the floor panting "or that was good" he said to himself. Normally I would grab my clothes and leg it upstairs as fast as I could. But I remained on the floor unable to move, suddenly William punched my arm and said "get your stuff and get a bath" I stood up picking my clothes up and walked calmly out of the front room as nothing had ever happened. I walked into the bathroom got into the bath, I washed and scrubbed myself all over with the brush after I had finished I put my nighty on, I had lost it. I was in world of my own, Arthur knew something was wrong that night and he bet it was all Williams fault, I laid down on my bed and pulled the covers tight around me (six weeks before my eleventh birthday I lost my virginity). I don't know if

I slept that night. But I do know one thing Arthur or my Lindsay could not help me now.

Arthur woke me in the morning very concerned with how I was; he kept on and on "what happened, what did he do?" I could not bring myself to tell him, felt dirty worthless and no more than a pieced of shit. I brushed him off and got dressed, as I walked down the stairs I had a feeling come over me, a strangeness that I have never felt before I was different, but not in a good way, I WAS SCUM, I was a used child. That bastard had changed my life forever and I had no say in it.

I was put on this earth to serve the adults purposes nothing else, so why did god give me a brain and feelings as well. This world is a very evil place, for a child I am supposed to be loved and cared for to be taught and shown the path of right and wrong, these words that we were told at school are all lies. I have now lost all my faith in everyone and everything.

School holidays were just great mother played her little games, and her new ones which was putting the sun chairs in the back garden and making Arthur and I sit in the full sun all-day with long trousers tops and thick jumpers on. Arthur and myself were both sick on the grass, on the first day of her new game, but that didn't stop her. Anyway our darling mother could think of punishing us she did. Her moods still went up and

down a lot she was what I think people call too faced.

William appeared no different, at meal times or in the evenings in the front room. He was also a very clever man Arthur and I started not to talk so much. For I even blamed the one person who loved me, for he was older than me bigger, taller, he was my big brother why could he not try at least to stop William. William did not leave any money in the bedroom anymore; he knew what I was doing (although he never said anything).

For the past two Mondays after brownies William had took me into the front room and raped me again, it got no better, the more he done it, the more withdrawn I got. I only had one more week of brownies and I just had to hold on to the fact after Monday he might just leave me alone. Do you know William is an occasional churchgoer? I often thought does he confess in his church, but I can't let myself think like that, because sometimes praying is all I have got left.

Arthur me and Mandy were all asleep one night when I suddenly woke up in terror, I sat and looked around the room, but mother was not waiting to pounce on me, instead I hear shouting its coming from downstairs. I crept out of bed made my way onto the upstairs landing Arthur was already there. There really going at each other Arthur said I sat next to him and together we tried to make out what they were saying, suddenly the

front room door burst open, Arthur and I legged it back to our bedrooms. William was shouting "and your no bloody wife your self" then we heard the front door slam shut, "shit" I said under my breath I pulled the bed covers tight up under my chin there will be no sleep tonight. There was banging and shouting going on downstairs what was she doing. I know Arthur would be listening and would be scared as well. Only Mandy slept on peacefully in her bed the noise stopped after about ten to fifteen minutes later, I think it was more frightening when it went all quiet for we didn't know where she was. Do you know when you try to listen so hard that you can not hear a bloody thing its like if you try and stare at something and your eyes water and you can not see? I had no watch there were no clocks upstairs I had no way of knowing the time, it seemed like hours that I was listening for (big mistake).

I awoke mother stood beside me "get your arse out of that bed and explain why you did it" she shouted at me "what, what"; I said getting out of bed. Mother grabbed my upper arm and pulled me into her room "destroy my things would you, write filth on my mirror I'll show you". I glanced at her dressing table the words upon it were wrote in lipstick across the mirror "MOTHERS A BITCH" just as I read it the first blow it me on the back of my head I fell to my knees beside her bed. Before I could put my hands on my head. Another one came down harder than the first. I cried out so loud. I thought even god himself would hear me.

But like every time before, I was in this hell just with mother, she beat me until I was black and blue all over, then she left me on her bedroom floor and went back downstairs, (for morning tea I suppose). Arthur crept in and sat beside me he was trying to stop me crying. For he knew if I didn't mother would return for some more Arthur helped me get up, and looking at my face he said "but in two days we go back to school your face its awful". "I don't care" I told him "I'll tell them all just what mother and William do to me". Arthur went to put his hand over my mouth but I pushed him away, I turned and grabbing hold of the banisters for support and walked into my room. Mandy lay in her bed asleep how the hell that kid slept through all the noise I don't know. It took me ages to get dressed my every movement was agony; she had beaten me with a pair of her shoes.

The next two days was hell, I just could not wait for Monday to come, to get away from mother, to start a new school, to be with my brother, all these things are good but it was also the last night of brownies and you know what that means.

It took ages to put on my new uniform, black skirt, white blouse, tie and a blazer and of course black shoes and a black bag. I looked good well except for the face but my note would explain that. I was still in a lot of pain on that first day of school. My note said and I said when asked "I fell over the handle bars of my bike whilst out

playing" great aye Arthur and me never even had a bike and as for going out playing "what was that?" but as always I had done what I was told.

There were classrooms everywhere, corridors everywhere, there were teachers all sorts of shapes and sizes good and bad ones I suppose when you get to know them. We didn't get to do a lot of work that first school day, but by the time I had arrived home I was totally knackered. My body was full of bruises if I only knew then what I know now I would be thankful for my bruises.

At dinner I said I felt sick when I didn't eat anything I was trying my best to get out of going to brownies but mother was having none of it. She went off to work I put my uniform on I just kept on telling myself that when he saw my broken body he would leave me alone. I didn't join in the party games that they were having that evening because half of my body was so full of bruises and it was painful the other half was that I was scared stiff of going home to William. I thanked Sally and her mum for taking and bringing me home each week and they said, "It was a pleasure".

William came to the front door as I walked through the stood in the hall and watched me take off my coat and shoes and put them away. I walked in silence along the hall and into the front room, William was behind me he closed the door and walked to the middle of the room. "Well come

on then you should know what to do by now". He undressed me like he always did. And I thought NOW's my chance I said "William look at my body please don't hurt me I am so sore" he looked me up and down and said "you will do" with that he grabbed me and pulled me down on the floor "the rest you know". He hurt me that night the worst he had done before, in my bath I swore to myself never again looking back I don't know what I was going to do, I just knew I could never let this happen again.

I dressed for the second day of school my brain and my mind was else where, I went in the bathroom to get washed and I caught a glimpse of myself in the mirror. I looked dead I don't think I was in my right mind but I saw Williams disposable razor on the window ledge and grabbed it and put it down my vest, without thinking I went downstairs to breakfast. Arthur kept on looking at me across the table but I pretended that I didn't notice.

Our journey to school was very quiet I didn't care just walked I had no plan or anything I just knew I had to stop it. I sat in the morning lesson pretending to work, but really I was not there. Lunchtime came I went and sat on the grass next to one of the playgrounds my mind was gone. The razor in my pocket I kept feeling with my hands, I looked around to see if anyone was looking and then I took it out and stood on it, it broke easy, just like me, I picked the blade up and returned it to my

pocket. The bell went soon after. Instead of going to my next lesson I went to the girl's toilets. I locked myself in a cubicle and removed my blazer. I rolled my sleeves up as far as they would go. And without thinking about it I started to slash the front of my arms, I felt no pain, again and again I cut them harder, harder my brain was saying, so harder I did it but still I felt no pain. When I had finished I felt a great sense of relief, in fact I felt the best I had ever felt since I could remember. I was not scared nothing mother or William has done came into my thoughts at all, I just felt relieved. I put the razor back in my bag and I picked up my blazer and left the girl's toilets. I can only imagine what I must have looked like, blood dripping from my hands, blood everywhere in fact, suddenly I heard a scream then more screams I stopped in my tracks, what's everyone screaming at. I didn't know well until an adult/teacher I think gently put an arm around me and led me to another corridor and into a small room. She sat down with me then she was talking to someone at the door, who, why, I didn't know, and I didn't care.

People came soon afterwards, lots of people but one I will never forget, they took me by car to another place, this one lady she was holding my arm and talking to me all the way. What she was saying I do not know, for I could see she was talking but I couldn't hear anything. They took me to a medical centre. And it was here that I had my first real cuddle. This lady (I never

knew her name) took off my blouse and cleaned both of my hands and arms up. She did this with such gentleness, (like I had never known before) she looked at me with such sadness in her eyes I liked her from that very moment, she bandaged my arms up I had done a good job. She then looked at my face and said something to me then pulled my vest up and then she saw my chest and then looked at my back, she gently lowered the vest and leant forward and cuddled me. I felt her warm body on mine and her strong arms holding me so gently, I felt I had died and gone to heaven. I stayed with her for a long time, I felt safe. My hearing came back and with it my feelings; my arms hurt really badly but to be with this lady to feel her warmth I would have done it again, any day.

She asked me who had done the bruising on my chest and back I could not answer her, I just sat and looked at her, she went to the door of the medical room and was talking don't know what about or to who, I didn't care. Later a man came to the door with tea for the lady and me. She asked me a lot of questions, but I could not tell her what she really wanted to know. "Who had hurt me"? I knew even on that first day, I could never tell a living soul, for Arthur was with them. This kind lady made me take off my vest so she could take photographs of my front, back, and face. I started to become frightened; I was not silly I knew something else was going on here. This lady went out of the room and within a few moments she

returned with a white tee-shirt and a red jumper, "come here child" she said to me lets get some clothes on you. I walked into her arms like I had never done to any adult before in my life, (well except Nan). I loved this lady she is mine I said to myself after she dressed me and sat together and started to drink our tea. I don't know what was going to happen and I didn't care, for I never wanted this time to ever end.

My lady as I call her now, kept on asking me who had hurt me? And why I had cut both my arms up? But I knew I had to remain silent. When we had finished our tea my lady asked if I could take my trousers and socks off, so she could take pictures of my legs. I didn't answer her at first but then I thought she has been so kind to me I can't see the harm in it. So slowly I stood up and undone the waist band and took my trousers off. Then my long socks and stood before her "oh you poor child" she said and I don't know why but all of a sudden I burst into tears, my lady once again cuddled me tight to her chest. Oh how I loved her. After the pictures had been taken, she asked "if I would remove my knickers". The minute she asked that I ran to the end of the room and squatted down with my arms around my knees and legs. "Leave me alone" I shouted at her. I want to go home, "now" said my lady coming towards me "no one is going to hurt you here Lindsay please believe me, we are trying to help. You don't have to do anything you don't want" "I want to get dressed I yelled at her" she said "fine"

if you come here I will help you" "I can do it myself" I replied, my lady watched me get dressed and I think she saw the pain I was in while it was being done.

Once dressed I sat on a small settee which was in a room, for I had done too much already. Mother would surely kill me for this; my lady went back to the door and started talking again. I slowly realised what trouble I was in. I sat shivering my arms hurt but I suppose no more than the rest of me. My lady came back in with another lady and a man, the minute I saw the man, (for he was old just like William) I jumped off the settee and ran to the corner of the room. I pulled a chair out from underneath the table and hid behind it. "I suspected this would happen". My lady told the others wait here, and she pulled the chair out a little bit and talked to me saying "no one was going to hurt you ever again" I knew that was not true, as she was so kind I came out and ran into her arms. "I need to in the car again," my lady said and holding my hand we all left the medical centre. I looked out of the window I didn't see anything, my mind was blank, and I didn't feel well, my stomach hurt and some sick come up in my mouth. I sat feeling really ill. At last the car stopped the other lady opened my door, as I rose to get out of the car my head went all fuzzy then nothing.

I awoke to my lady sitting on a bed, a bed that I was in she talked gently to me saying "you

fainted" what ever that is. I was at a children's home not far from my home and that I was to stay here for a while I didn't know how long. I looked around the room there was a wardrobe, a chest of drawers, a mirror and a bed. Oh and a window, my lady told me its alright here that I would like it here and I said "but what about Arthur" "It's ok she replied we are going to sort all that out you don't have to worry about anything". After about half an hour my lady left she left me with a lady called Mary she was dressed funny, and she had long fair hair (really long) and her clothes were different she had these great big beads around her neck but she looked nice. I didn't ask any questions for I didn't care what happened to me. Being away from mother and William was enough. I spent the next two days wandering around. Keeping my ears to the ground as they say "there was a lot of children here" all ages boys and girls alike it was like a massive house with lots of children the people who the house belonged to the children called auntie Mary and uncle Dave. They had a flat joined on down stairs, then there was Auntie Wendy and uncle Alan, they had a flat upstairs, they had a kid, a boy younger than me don't know his name yet. All the children had their own rooms, there was a large kitchen a dinning room and a big playroom with a television and a big fish tank in it and the best thing was that everyone could play with the toys whenever they liked. Also probably the best thing was that there was a long driveway with big gates. (So people couldn't get in) and under a roof next to the kitchen there were bikes,

small ones, and big ones also there was skate boards, go-carts, skipping ropes and footballs and we could play with them all as long as it was not raining. My children's home was the best any kid could wish for and I was so grateful to be here. The only downfall that I had was that my brother was not here with me.

Auntie Mary came to my room Thursday afternoon; she knocked on the door before she entered. She asked me "if I felt any better". I replied "yes thank you". She asked if there was anything that I wanted to ask. I said no. Then she told me that in the morning she would be taking me to Milton to see a psychiatrist. "Why" I asked. She said "because of what you did to your arms" that was not normal we are worried that you need help and someone to talk to. I looked at her and said quite loudly "I am not mad you know". "Lindsay" she said, "no one said you are" that's not what a psychiatrist is for, liar I thought. Auntie Mary stayed with me for a while, but I remained angry I will show them I thought. The two days or rather nights I had been here I had slept like a log my body was healing, but my arms are still bad Auntie Wendy had put clean bandages on today I am glad you didn't need stitches she said. Do you know at dinner times we all sit in the dinning room and we can talk and eat any way we like? Things here are so different in the time I have been here I have seen no kid getting hit, no adult getting angry, it was like I had been transferred to another world, but yes I still miss my brother.

At ten o'clock the next morning Auntie Mary and I were taken by taxi to a child clinic about ten minutes away. I felt nervous because of what he or she would ask me. I had to stick to what I had worked out in bed. A man came out of one of the doors and called my name out, Auntie Mary Rose and I followed the man into his office. He explained who he was. And that he only wanted to help, he spoke very gentle for a man and made me feel at ease very quickly, he took some notes from Auntie Mary and asked her to undo one of my arms so he could see for him self what I had done. As Auntie Mary was undoing my left arm I saw the doctor, what ever his name was looking at some pictures "oh my god" I suddenly felt my heart start beating very fast I'm in trouble what now, my arm lay on my lap for all to see. I looked at it and thoughts went darting through my head. The doctor came around to my side of the table and had a look at my arm, asking Auntie Mary "is the other one the same" she nodded and started to redress my arm. When she had finished the doctor asked for her to wait outside as she rose from her chair, I also went to get up the doctor assured me that I would be quite safe with him and that Auntie Mary would only be outside.

He talked a lot, saying that children who had been hurt by their mothers or fathers sometimes blamed themselves. And the children were not to blame. He asked why I had cut my arms up and he waited for my reply. I just said, "I

don't know". For that was the truth, he asked where did you get the razor from, so I told him, then he said, "Why did you take the razor if you had not intended to cut yourself?" I had no answer and that was the truth.

Over the weekend I was told that I had to start back at school on Monday, I was to get a bus and they would show me where to get on for school and where to catch it back again. Auntie Mary could see the fear that had risen in my eyes and continued quickly saying that I was to remain at the children's home. "Great" I will see Arthur at school but to return to the children's home afterwards, at last my life was starting to get better.

Our first meeting was very tearful, for we had both missed each other so very much, mother had told him nothing, even my name was not to be spoken, he heard about my arms and the blood from school. I really felt for him because, there was me having fun and he was still with them, thinking all sorts of things had happened, anyway we were together again now and we enjoyed each others company. Things remained the same for about a month. I had found a new way of life and it was great, I was learning to ride a bike, it was really hard but fun. Do you know that the sun shines over the children's home all day and the birds sing? I could lie on my bed and hear them, everything in my life was just brilliant, I felt so lucky, and then the bombshell was dropped. It was

Thursday; I had just finished my homework when there was a knock on my door. Auntie Mary came in and I could tell straight away that something was wrong, she sat on my bed and explained that by law they couldn't stop my parents from seeing me, and that they had agreed that one weekend in four, I was to return home. I just sat there; I didn't know what to say. How could they do this to me, I have been so good, I have not done anything wrong, Auntie Mary explained to me that on Friday after school I was to go home and not to return back here. My parents would bring me back by six on Sunday, she then carried on saying something about a care order, but I had heard enough. My mind went blank. I never slept a wink that night, why had this happened, my lady told me that I would never have to see them again. "Didn't anyone realise what they were doing to me?" Didn't anyone care? (Course I realised now, I never told a soul of what mother or William was doing to me, so how could they know), but they had the pictures, they must have known that I couldn't have done all that to myself. I was sure my lady knew what was going on, or did she? Did she also think that I had done all my injuries myself, over and over in my head I had tried to (play back) what had happened that day, but there was so many blanks, I couldn't make sense of it all. Anger started to creep into my body as I lay in my bed, I loved her, I thought she understood, all she said were lies, I hit my fist against my wall again and again in fact until I looked up and there was blood on the wall. I stared at my open hand "I

felt nothing", I got up out of bed and put some toilet paper around my hand (it was lose on the chest of drawers) I then returned back to my bed. I was angry, but also scared, well not yet but that would come tomorrow, I lay thinking, even that psychiatrist bloke, but I had not told him anything, just like my lady and Auntie Mary but now I wanted to <u>live</u> not die. My anger stayed with me for the best part of the night, and then I suppose I talked myself into the fact it was only one weekend in four.

I had managed for eleven years, so I could do this, but also it was a weekend so mother didn't go to work, so we was not alone with William. Plus I could be with Arthur and Mandy. I had to keep thinking like this for I was strong now. Both in mind and body. I could do this. I calmed myself down and realised by now my hand was throbbing. I unwound the toilet paper and stared at my hand. "Bloody hell" had I done that, all my knuckles were cut also the palm of my hand, I crept out of bed and went down the hall to the bathroom (there was four of them upstairs). I washed gently for it hurt quite a bit; I dried it and returned to my room. After a few minutes I got back in bed, I lay awake trying to clear my mind. All of a sudden without me trying I was in Lindsay's room with her, this has never happened before, I always had to concentrate before, "I was shocked", but glad if you know what I mean, we talked, it was so easy for she knew everything.

I sat on <u>her</u> floor next to her and like every time before a sense of peace and calm came over me. (I suppose it was like some people think heaven, would be) Lindsay's room had a door, a white one, but you could miss it quite easily for it just blended in with the walls for there was no handle or key hole, nothing. The walls were as white as snow with no windows, no entrance, even the floor was white, you could call it a box, but we were safe and happy together we could have been anywhere, as long as we was <u>ONE</u>. We talked, mostly I talked and Lindsay listened, but the senses of calm overcame me so I just sat back and relaxed. (It's funny but I never once questioned how she could be me and how I could be me in two different places).

I walked around school in a daze that day, only Arthur over the moon. At home time he was at the gate waiting for me. As we walked I told him more about my children's home, I asked him how he was getting on with mother, he explained, that he thought when I had left home, he would get the beatings but so far he had remained safe. Looking at my brother as he talked, I realised he was growing up so fast, I thanked God for that. Our weekend passed with no beatings. The house still felt the same, mother was still the same but it felt like she wanted to explode but couldn't. We never set foot outside the house all weekend, well only in the back garden to brush our hairs.

At 5.30pm on Sunday, Mother went upstairs. I was praying for the next half-hour to pass quickly. But about five minutes later mother came back down the stairs with a dustbin bag tied at the top. She threw it by the front door, William announced it was time to be going and told us to put our coats and shoes on and to wait outside by his car. Arthur and I did as we were told. Outside I cuddled Arthur and gave him a kiss, he had tears in his eyes "I'll see you tomorrow at school" I said, he turned and wiped his face with the sleeve of his coat "poor Arthur I feel sorry for him". William drove Arthur and me back to the children's home, we sat in the back holding hands and we both knew what each other was thinking. On our arrival William pulled up outside the big gates. He got out and walked passed my door to the boot of the car; I kissed my brother and got out. William threw the dustbin bag at my feet and said "you will be needing these" he then turned and opened his door, got in, and drove away. I stood and watched Williams car go up the road, Arthur was staring out of the back window I watched them until they were out of sight, then I picked up my bag and went inside. Everything was the same as I had left it on Friday morning, why I thought it would be any different I don't know. In my room I emptied the black bin bag onto my bed, and stood and stared at them. Clothes all clothes, nothing else, (well I had nothing else, so what else I thought there would be I don't know).

I settled back down to my new life in the children's home. I started to play on my own, and with others it didn't matter. I also did not fear the two Uncles that lived with us anymore even. Dr Patel my shrink - whom I visited once a month. But there was something that was starting to happen to me that got me worried it was so hard to explain, I was riding on the scooter in the drive way, when mother shouted at me to get off it, I stopped and froze in my tracks. I looked all around. No one, I stood for a few minutes, thinking she must be hiding somewhere. I was shaking with fear. I don't know how long I stood in the driveway. But I tell you this I was frightened. Also again one night a few weeks later I had a nightmare. I awoke to mother yelling at me, I stared at her face, and her eyes were black (all black) I screamed like I had never screamed before, and suddenly I was slapped across my face. As my eyes opened wider I could see Auntie Mary leaning over me, with both arms I grabbed for her and pulled her down on top of me, I sobbed my heart out for hours after that. Auntie Mary kept on saying "it's just a bad dream, it's not real, and you're safe". (For if she only knew) I had no more sleep, in that night, for something was happening that I could not control.

As time went on I continued to go home every one weekend in four, although, I had no beatings, or sexual abuse, they were frightening times. Mandy and Arthur had both grown so much, my room was just like a strangers, all that

remained of <u>me</u> was the bed, and the teddy Nan had given me as a baby on one of the shelves. Dinner times, in fact, anytime I was spoken to and treated like a piece of shit. I didn't care, for I was just so grateful for my children's home and my new life there.

More time than I would like to remember. I heard my mother's voice, always shouting or yelling at me. It was not like Lindsay, for I went to her on my own accord, and could leave the same way. But mother, I never knew when her voice would come. (Eating dinner, having a bath, talking, sleeping or playing) I had no control, just like I never had, it was hard, I was on guard again, but I started to realise that all though, I could hear mothers voice, I couldn't see her, and believe you and me, I did look for her. What was going on I didn't know, but I knew I had to keep it to my self.

Since my new life began and I was fit again. I started to enjoy my p-e lessons at school a great deal. For I found out that I could run, <u>really run</u>. Twice a week our p-e teacher Miss Bunting would do outside p-e with us, netball, hockey, track running, and my favourite, cross country running, I don't mean to sound big headed, but I was winning all the time, and the buzz I got from it, was out of this world. For I was good at something, I began to try and make myself better; I would run everywhere every chance I had. About a month or so later the school sports day was coming, after p-e, one day Miss Bunting took me

aside and said "I wanted to enter you for the cross country and the four hundred flat what do you think?" "Yes" I replied, without even thinking I felt so proud, someone believed in me, at home that night I told Auntie Mary about my day, she was over the moon. I started to walk around with my head up, not down all the time. Two weeks later at school, Miss Bunting wanted me to stay behind because she wanted a word, Miss Bunting sat me down and started to explain that an ex-trainer that had retired would like to come and see me run. "Why?" I said, because Lindsay you are an exceptional runner and with more help than I can give you, you could really go places. "But I live in a children's home" I said, I know, I have phoned them, and explained everything and have given me permission for you to stay back after school for one hour twice a week, and they agreed, and as long as I was supervising you as well. I sat and looked at her, I didn't know what to say I thought two people, one I didn't even know are willing to help me "why?". Miss Bunting could see I was having a hard time taking it all in. She touched my arm, and looked right into my eyes and said "you're good, really good and we can make you better" give it a try you have got nothing to lose, I stood up and replied "thank you for believing in me. I won't let you down". On my way home on the bus, her words were going over and over in my head, I walked into the home with my head up high in the clouds.

In my room after dinner I could not get to Lindsay in her room quick enough. I sat beside her and told her word for word what had been said. I was so happy; I thought to myself I was good at running, because I had spent my whole life running from mother. I spent a long time with Lindsay that evening and I had noticed something that I had not realised before, "I looked older than her", was it just me, was I just seeing things that were not really there, maybe.

Two day's later on my p-e day. Miss Bunting introduced me to a grey hair fit, old man. Mr Roberts. He shook my hand and said, "He would like to see me run". I liked him straight away. He talked kind, and his big hand was so gentle when he shook mine. It was our lesson so with the rest of my class we lined up for the cross country track, I felt a bit nervous because I knew he would be watching me, but I knew I had to give it all I had got. OFF the whistle went and I ran. I ran, for <u>me</u>, in and out of my schoolmates. Into the woods through the trees my legs were just taking me. My heart was pumping like never before. Exited the woods, jumped over the stile and round the track on the first big field. My head, looking forward and I ran like the wind. "I felt free" the first field ran. I turned sharp left into the dirt track. Mud was flying up all over me. But I kept on running, at least I could see the last field, my heart was beating ten to a dozen, I glanced behind me, no one, I turned back and with every ounce of strength I had I bolted for the finish line. "I won". I said to myself as I flopped onto the ground. Mr

Roberts and Miss Bunting were coming my way, I sat on my bum panting heavily, but my heart was full of joy. As they approached I got to my feet, waiting to see what they had to say. I noticed that they both had stop watches in their hands. "Not bad" Mr Roberts said, "but you could do better, you know with my help" "but I won" I said feeling a bit down hearted "yes" said Mr Roberts, but you had no real competition, wait until the regional finals. That's the test. I looked at my teacher and she could see I didn't really understand. "What had been said, Lindsay" she said "the school has a big p-e day once a year, I am putting you in for the cross-country and the four hundred metres, we know you will win <u>both</u> easily". Then about two weeks after that all the winners from the schools all over Essex is coming <u>here</u> for the grand finals. That's what Mr Roberts means we need to get you fit and ready and the fastest you can be, for that's "our goal for all of us to aim for". I stood and looked at them both and I thought to myself "no one has wanted me to win at anything before; no one has ever tried to help me to want to better myself before". I will do as they say and maybe one day I might even make someone proud of me. "Hit the showers" Miss Bunting said and Mr Roberts shouted "see you straight after school with your kit on Tuesdays and Thursdays, don't be late".

As I showered my mind was going mad, I kept on thinking if could win these races then I would not be useless, stupid, dirty, good for

nothing bitch anymore. Maybe mother would be proud of me, and leave my head forever; it was worth a try.

Chapter Seven

As predicted I did win both races, I was given two gold coloured coins in boxes. I was so proud of myself. I couldn't wait for the bus to take me home that afternoon. I was eager to show Auntie Mary my coins. I stood before her in the kitchen as she studied my wins, her face told me she was very pleased and so did her words, I never felt this good before ever. I ran to my room for I had to tell Lindsay, it took ages to find her in my mind because I was so excited (I suppose. When you try and do anything in a hurry it takes longer). I showed Lindsay my coins I told her blow for blow about each of my races she kept on telling me to slow down, after I had told her everything even what Auntie Mary had said I sat back next to her and felt a sudden relief come over me. Suddenly I heard a noise I opened my eyes and Auntie Mary was in my room. "Oh no I thought how long had she been there". By the look in her eyes long enough "Lindsay who have you been talking too? When I came in your room there was no one but yet you were holding a conversation with someone, what's going on?" I stared at her not knowing what to say, for I had been found out, but Lindsay was mine and no one could ever find out about her. I looked Auntie Mary straight in the eyes and said "I was talking to myself I do it when I am a bit lonely". As she left my room she turned and looked back at me, as if to say you're lying. I knew from now on. I had to

be very careful. No one must ever find out about my Lindsay.

Tomorrow was Thursday good p e after school, but it also this weekend that I had to return home. I always saw Arthur at dinnertime; for all though we had both grown up a lot since I left home we were still very close. He had seen me win both of my races. I had brought my coins into school today, so I could show him "well done sis" he said "I'm so proud of you". Those words were like a million dollars to me. I told him all about Mr Roberts. And after school and dinner time running, he told me "to go for it" we parted before the bell went so I walked around to the back of my school and put my bags and coat down, and decided to run a lap of the track. I started to run then. I had to stop. And kick off my shoes. Then off again I ran. The wind blew through my hair, I lifted my head right up straight it felt grand, that is the moment the voice hit me "**YOU CANT RUN STOP IT YOU STUPID BITCH**" I stopped dead in my tracks and stood like a soldier to attention. I looked all around, every direction; there was no one. I said out loud. "I don't have to do as you say anymore". No answer came, I repeated my words again, but this time louder, suddenly her voice came again "**YOU LITTLE SLUT YOU GOOD FOR NOTHING YOURE WORSE THAN USELESS YOURE PATHETIC**". These were her words being shouted at me; I ran to my things, grabbed them and ran for the school. I hid in the girl's toilets, I was out of breath, and panting my heart beating

so fast I thought I would die. I sat on the toilet trying to calm myself down, when I noticed under the toilet roll holder there were two cigarettes and a book of matches, I pulled the tape away that held them in place. I had never smoked in my life, but now, I thought it would calm me down. I had seen kids do it; it didn't look hard. I lit the fag, err it was foul, but I made myself carry on with it, after about half of the fag I threw it down the pan and tapped the other one back up. I returned to class feeling quite sick. I didn't do my work that afternoon, for all I could think about was mother. I was seeing her this weekend I would try and do something about it, what I didn't know. By the end of the day, my sickness had gone when I went to get changed for my running. Miss Bunting and Mr Roberts were waiting for me on the field. I ran to them both and started warming up the way Miss Bunting had shown us all in lesson. Mr Roberts came over and told me that I could knock seconds off my time if I did a block start; he had put one out at the one hundred-metre race. We all walked to the start and Mr Roberts got down and went through the different positions for using it. I copied him, not very well at first, but like he said the more I try the better I would get. We had a lot of starting of races. At each one I was getting better. We did a one hundred-metre flat race with blocks and one without them. I was three seconds quicker with the blocks, for Mr Roberts was right, after the hour I was knackered and glad to be going home, on the bus it dawned on me that I would be going home for the weekend tomorrow. In bed during the night

I was again woken by noise, I lay waiting for fear it was of who it was, moments later Uncle Dave popped his head around my door, I gasped "its alright Lindsay I'm only doing my nightly rounds, why are you not asleep?" "I had dream" I replied, "are you alright now?" "Yes" I replied as my door was closed. I lay awake for a long time thinking about mother, did I have the guts to say anything to her, I didn't know, but I will just have to see how she is.

As always my darling brother was waiting at the gate for me. He smiled as I approached, "come on the best runner in the school" he shouted to me, I'm sure I went red, we talked all the way home just like old times, mother had started to have bad moods again, Arthur told me to be very careful this weekend. Apparently she shouted a lot at William these days, my heart really bled for the man, but even so I knew that Arthur was serious and I would take his warning with heed. As we entered the front door I could feel bad vibes, or something. We remained safe that night, for as Arthur had said it was William she was after not us, (it felt really good that my bastard of a stepfather was getting some punishment for a change). Saturday, Arthur, Mandy and I were allowed to play in the playroom quietly we were all just great full to be out the way, I asked Arthur what was wrong with mother he didn't really know, but it had been going on for quite a while. I looked at Mandy; she was growing up so fast and Arthur, well he was nearly as tall as

mother and his stutter were nearly gone. Do you know that I thought my little Arthur is growing into a fine looking young man?

After dinner we went to watch TV for a while, William was with us, just like he was trying to hide, for once in my life I hope mother wins, maybe William should get a taste of what it was like being on the other end of the stick. Mother was in the kitchen making a hell of a racket. We were told to go and get our nightclothes on we obeyed promptly. I went with Mandy into our room to get undressed. She asked me if I would undress her, and I obeyed, for I knew all she wanted was a warm touch. She went back down. And I started to undress myself, as I pulled my knickers down; I stared at them with disbelief. They were full of blood, I ran to the bathroom and scrubbed them in the basin, (most of it came out but not all) I kept wiping myself with the toilet paper but more and more blood, just kept on coming. I think I knew what it was I had heard girls at school talking, but what do I do to <u>stop it,</u> I put a clean pair of knickers on and rolled some toilet paper up and put that between my legs. I needed them towel things, I looked in the mirror in the bathroom, my face was as white as a sheet, I walked downstairs hoping my toilet paper wouldn't fall out. Mother was still in the kitchen; I approached her, but she just pushed straight passed me and went into the dinning room. I decided to stay were I was, I was very nervous, I would have rather told Mr Roberts than to have to confront mother.

100

Mother came back in. "This is my big chance" I thought. I went up to her and just about to open my mouth. When, again she pushed me aside and went through the hall. "Shit" I said to myself. I went into the downstairs toilet. And put fresh toilet paper in. Again, I waited in the kitchen for mother to return. And sure enough carrying two cups she walked straight pass me to the sink. "Shit or bust I thought" I walked up to mother and tried to explain to mother what was wrong, "oh got the curse have you", there is some tampons in the cupboard in the toilet, use them, and she waved me off just like she was the queen. I locked myself in the toilet and opened the cupboard, I looked and looked tampons, tampons, and I kept on saying to myself for I didn't know what they were. On the bathroom shelf there was two long things, I picked one up and on the outside it said super tampon, thank god I thought, I took it out of the wrapper there was cotton wool with a string inside this long tube. No instructions nothing, no box, what the bloody hell do I do with it, tears started to roll down my cheeks as panic set in, I had been in the toilet a long time, mother would be after me soon if I did not hurry up. I pulled the white cord and the cotton wool came out of the holder. I stood with it in my hands feeling totally bloody useless, in the end I put it down the toilet, and wrapped some more toilet paper up for my knickers; I would just lie, and keep on doing this until I got back to the children's unit. Where I know I would get the help I needed.

I took my place on the end of the settee and looked forward to bedtime. For two hours mother, William, Arthur and I sat in pure silence. Mandy was taken to bed by William a lot earlier, I don't know if it was my imagination, but my legs and bum felt wet, I prayed to myself that I had not come through, for my nighty was white and dressing gown cream. I knew I could not move for I had not been told too. I just sat and hoped that god was on my side for once. Finally later than usual mother told us to go to bed, I stood up and tried to edge my way to the door for it was better to be safe than sorry. Arthur walked through and as I followed I heard mother give out the most awful scream. I froze; she jumped out of her chair and flew across the room. **"YOU DIRTY FILTHY HOAR"** she screamed at me. She grabbed my hair and pulled me through the door and into the kitchen. With one almighty blow she had me on the floor. Screaming and shouting. All the time is pulling things out of the cupboard under the sink. I half sat up and was trying to tell her I did not know what to do with her tampons. When again she hit me across the face, not with her hand but with a brush. I heard William shouting, he was telling her "not to hurt me". But she just threw a yellow bottle of something right at him. And he disappeared through the door. "Stand up she told me, stand you slut". I began to get myself up but it was not quick enough for her, because again she grabbed a handful of my hair and pulled so hard a big clump of it came out in her hand. My mother then

ripped (and I mean ripped) my nighty and dressing gown from my back. I stood before her in my knickers. My eye was already closing, where it had got the full force of one of her blows. **"TAKE YOU'RE KNICKERS OF YOU PROSTITUTE"** she said to me. As I did the toilet paper fell on to the floor, mother saw it and bent down to pick it up. She then rubbed it in my face. Mother hit me again around the head and again I fell to the floor as I lay there feeling dizzy, I could hear mother shouting and clattering about what was she doing God above only knows. Mother grabbed my legs and laid me flat on the kitchen floor. Then with the hard floor brush and vim I think. She started scrubbing it in between my legs. I yelled with pain but it made no difference. She picked up a blue bottle and started to pour it all over my private parts, the brush was hard. She was hard. I screamed and screamed. She turned me over like a rag doll, and then she scrubbed all my bottom and upper legs. I had never felt <u>pain</u> like it before; I went through absolute hell. How could a mother put her child through this I thought it would never end, but thanks to William, for I heard him saying **"WHAT THE HELL HAVE YOU DONE"**. Stop it you bitch get off her, I felt mother being pulled off me.

I think I must have passed out, because all I can remember was William drying me and then carrying me up to my bed, the rest is blank. I woke while it was dark tears streaming down my swollen face and yet I was not crying, for I would never cry

again. I tried to get out of bed but my head and my eyes went all hazy. I lay thinking to myself; mother had hurt me all my life. For as long as I can remember but this, was pure evil, my whole middle section was scrubbed raw, I felt under the bed clothes and I was wearing something, I felt with my hands all around my privates, it was a nappy. I was sure of it but you know I didn't even care.

I was ordered by William to stay in bed until I had to go back, for that I was very grateful. Arthur came up to see me that day and he brought me a packet of sanitary towels, William had sent him up to the corner shop with a note for them. Arthur looked at me with tears running down his cheeks. I told him not to worry and that I would be alright when I got back to the home. I put my hand on his arm and said very calmly. "Watch out for your self she is mad" he leant over the bed and gave a kiss to my forehead, I love you sis <u>always</u>. And with that he was gone. I lay on my bed and I knew that I had to do something, but what, if it wasn't for Arthur I would tell the world what had gone on in this house. But that was not an option, I protected him all my life, I would not stop now or put him in danger. I had no way of knowing what the time was; I got up and went to the bathroom with my knickers and a sanitary towel. I rolled the bloody nappy up. I put my knickers and a towel on and it really hurt. It was my first look at what she had done to me. Oh my god, you don't want to know I thought, I was raw there was blisters all

over my legs, privates, lower belly and the back I could not see, but I think it was the same, it hurt really bad. Just having knickers on, for I dreaded getting dressed but I knew I had to so I could get the hell out of here; I took the dirty nappy back into my room and started to dress myself. It was nothing short of pure agony. I cried the whole time, but not out loud only to myself, for no one was going to hurt me again. (I don't know how I knew it I just did). Arthur came upstairs and into my room just as I had finished. He told me that William had sent him up to tell me that we were leaving in ten minutes. I waved Arthur to come near to me. I looked my brother straight in the eyes and told him, "that what ever happened I loved him with every breath of my body, and always would". He replied with a tone in his voice that I had not heard before, "don't be silly sis". As he was walking out of my door. I asked. "Is mother coming"? He said. "No William told her she better stay behind". I packed my things and slowly very slowly, edged my way downstairs. William came into the hall put his coat and shoes on and opened the front door to unlock his car. All of a sudden I remembered my teddy on the shelf in my bedroom. I couldn't leave it for Nan and Granddad had bought for me when I was a baby. I asked Arthur to run up and get it, I told him to be quick, he returned and we both rammed the teddy in my bag. We walked out the front door and as I closed it behind me I had one last look at the house of hell and quite loudly said, "Fuck you" and closed the door got into the car with Arthur. On our

journey we held hands as we always did, but it was a lot more intense than normal, I feared for him, at least he was bigger now, more able if need be to defend himself. When we arrived it took me a lot longer than normal to get out of Williams's car, I waited as I always did and watched my brothers head facing away as the car left my sights. I picked up my bag and headed for the back door that led into the kitchen, I walked straight through the kitchen, I heard Auntie Mary or Wendy calls my name but I did not respond. I walked straight into the dinning room, dropped my bag picked up a dinning room chair and preceded to the TV room. I walked straight up to the big glassfish tank and raised the chair high up into my arms and smashed it straight down into the tank. Water poured out soaking me completely I stood like a statue with half a chair still in my hands, as voices about me was screaming and shouting, shapes kept on moving in front of me then I felt people holding me trying to prise my hands open. I could do nothing. For I think I was catatonic or like it. Next I remember both Aunties undressing me for I was soaked through. As they removed my bottom half of clothes. I heard gasps from them. I heard one of them say something about a doctor. They laid me in my bed naked and Auntie Mary sat in my room with me, no words were exchanged for I couldn't speak, that I wanted to. All I could think about was Arthur.

Five days later Auntie Mary said. "I just woke up". She questioned me on and off all that

day about my injuries. I was as usual silent. The doctor had visited me twice while I lay in my bed. I had like a netting stuff and padding all over my middle body. Auntie Mary told me to be careful when I went to the toilet. And that a nurse would be coming to put clean dressings on. I felt sorry for Auntie Mary, she tried so hard to get me to talk if only I could tell her, but Arthur still had to be protected and I was not at home anymore this was the only way of protecting him.

The nurse came the following day and was appalled at my injuries, she was very nice and gentle as she changed my dressings, although I must admit I did feel a bit embarrassed but I was at that age. As the nurse was packing up to leave. There was a knock at my bedroom door, the nurse opened it and Auntie Mary came in and behind her Dr Patel, "hello Lindsay" he said "I have come to see you for a change". Alarm bells started ringing in my head something was up. Auntie Mary and the nurse left, leaving my bedroom door open. Dr Patel sat on my chest of drawers and started talking to me; he was very concerned about my mental state about the violence but most of all my five days of lack of response as he called it, and not forgetting my injuries. I listened to him and all the time I kept on saying in my head "leave me alone, leave me alone" at first because I did not talk he left me, to think about things and to call him if I wanted to talk. Joke aye.

Alone in my room, I felt knackered, my body was healing my face was nearly better when could I return to school, I didn't know, but I knew Arthur would be really worried. I decided to make an effort to get back too normal, I left my room and made my way downstairs. In the TV room there was no fish tank, it looked bare, I felt guilty, so I walked through the dinning room and into the kitchen. Two of the other kids were in there getting a drink. They started whispering and grinning. I knew it was about me. I threw the cup I had got ready for my drink. And shouted at them that if they had something to say, "Then say it". Carol the oldest looked at me and said. "We all hate you, you killed all the fish you're a murderer" the words ran through me with such guilt, I couldn't say anything for it was true I had killed them all. I turned and ran back to my safe place, I felt so bad, I hadn't planned to kill the bloody fish, but that didn't make what I had done right. I mean I didn't like fish very much but I would never have harmed them "well not normally".

Auntie Mary came into the room and said "that we had to have a really serious talk" something was really wrong I knew by the tone of her voice.

I was moved to a psychiatric children's unit in Patterson, north Yorkshire, they would be more equipped to meet my needs "but Arthur" I said its alright she said you will still see him "but what about school?" I asked, "There is a school

attached to the unit". Lindsay this home can not cope with your violent outbursts, it's not fair on the other children and on you, there you will get the help you need, "but I will miss you" and we will miss you too but we can write you know. Now there is something else the home has applied for, a full care order to be paced on you some time ago and because of what happened last week, Dr Patel got it pushed through quicker. I stared at her not understanding what she was talking about Auntie Mary looked at my face and knew she would have to explain further. Lindsay, we all feel you have been an abused child. The pictures we have of when you first came to us and the injuries you have now, all the nightmares and a lot of things but because you have never told us anything, we feel all we can do is to put this order on you and protect you. We can not make whoever did these things "pay". I thought about what she was saying and realised again MOTHER HAD WON. I was moving further away from my brother and I would not see him at school when would I be moving I asked Auntie Mary, quietly she said tomorrow. I gasped "but Arthur I need to tell him, indeed to see him please I need to see my brother".

"It won't be possible well not yet anyway", "why?" I asked pleading "because the care order forbids any contact with your family Lindsay" she said, "you have got to understand we are just trying to protect you. I think you have been through hell in your short life, believe me we are

only trying to help you." Tears rolled down my face like a stream running into a waterfall. Auntie Mary left my room. And sobbing became uncontrollable, all I ever cared about was my brother Arthur he was my life my reason for living and now we was going to be parted and all for my good so they say. Around and around what Auntie Mary had said went through my head didn't matter what I did, MOTHER had won. I bet she planned all of this, just to get rid of me forever; well she would not win for I could leave north Yorkshire and see my brother any time I wanted. (What I didn't know was it was one hundred and fifty miles away). I lay on my bed and tried to think of good things, I only came up with two. Number one, I would not ever have too see mother again number two, William as well. The more I said these to myself the happier I made myself, but always in my mind was my darling brother. It's like I always had a purpose in life, to protect him from mother now I could not do it but I assured myself within a week I would be laughing and joking with him.

Ten thirty the next morning a man named Steve King was introduced to me by Auntie Mary she explained he was my court appointed social worker and he was taking me to Patterson where the children's unit was. I looked at him (actually he was good looking) and he picked up my bags "is that all" he asked "yes" I replied with that Auntie Mary took my hand and led me into the kitchen. Uncle Dave, Auntie Wendy and Uncle Alan and a few of the children was there too. Uncle Dave

gave me a present and told me to be good and to look after my self they said they would all miss me I said my good byes and Auntie Mary took me out to the car. I hugged her with feelings I never knew I had then I got into Steve's car and started off to begin my new life.

I fell asleep and when I woke the car was stopped outside these big metal gates, Steve had his window down and was talking into this box. I rubbed my eyes; this can't be right, looks like a bloody prison. Suddenly the big metal gates opened. Steve drove the car in. When I looked behind us the gate was closing. "Where the hell are we?" I shouted at Steve. "Hey it's all right we are here, the children's unit". Steve got out of the car so I followed him. He got my bags out of the boot and told me to follow him to the door. I was petrified the door was unlocked by a big fat lady. She was foreign. She spoke funny. But Steve understood her because we followed her down this small corridor and into a small room she said something, and left I could hear the sound of children in the background, I turned to Steve with a worrying look he just said it's alright but some of the kids here are really ill. Well that really made me feel better. A man came and welcomed me. And told me he was the boss, Mr Manner, and that someone would show me my bed and explain the rules. The two men exchanged papers and talked. But I could not hear what they were saying. At that moment the big fat lady walked straight up to me, just about stopping herself right in my face, she shouted something, picked my bags and started

walking further down a long hall I followed her with fear in my heart I was scared.

We walked into a massive room like a hospital ward. Beds on both sides, lockers, and the curtain that had to be pulled around each one. She was saying something but her English was so bad I could only understand bits of it. We got about three-quarters of the way down and she stopped. I think this was my bed. Yes it must be because she threw my bags on the bed she pointed to the chair and shouted something; I sat my butt on that chair and thought my life had come to an end.

A bit later a lady was making her way down the line of beds towards me, she had keys hanging on a chain on her belt, she sat on my bed and began to go through the rules of the unit, maybe life would not be so bad after all. Only the front door was locked and the gates to the car park in front of the unit. We had pocket money each week and there was a tuck shop there so we could spend it. The school adjoined the unit at the back. They liked children to go but would not make us (wow great no school) we had set times for everything a buzzer sounded so we all knew when meal times were, the only thing was the fact I didn't have my own room. A lady told me I would soon get used to sleeping like it the top half was the boys then half way down there was shutters then the bottom half was for the girls. The ladies name was Beth she told me to unpack and she would come and get me to show me around. I obeyed her every word. As good as her word she

was back and talking me through every room. It was a big place it held up to eighteen kids and they always had six staff on duty day and night. Beth went on to explain that life was never quiet here, for the kids were very disturbed also that they often use drugs on kids that got out of control. I was learning a whole different way of life. The TV room was big really big. So was the dinning room. There were kids hanging around in both. Then Beth took me to the school, well that wasn't much then we went out of the back door into a massive garden. There were tyre swings, a climbing frame, logs that you could walk on, football net, a see saw and at the other end a basket ball net. Beth could see that I was impressed "you are all allowed out here when ever you like" she said. We walked back in and a boy was sitting on the washing machine with a hand puzzle of some sort. Beth introduced us his name was Billy. He looked about my age Beth just told me to wander around by myself for tea would be in half-hour or so. I took myself to the TV room; a cartoon was on the box. The clock on the wall said four thirty five, but that could not be right. We left at ten thirty am. We have only been here an hour to hour and a half at the most, I got up and walked into the kitchen, the clock in there said the same I felt panic set in, I tried to find Beth. I needed someone for all the clocks was wrong. I found my way to the first hall I shouted for Beth I shouted again and again. In my anger I picked up a chair and started swinging it around out of nowhere adults appeared. "Beth" I shouted. "The clocks, all

the clocks are wrong." Beth tried to calm me down. But I had worked myself up into such a frenzy that even my words were not making sense. The adults were all closing in on me. I just kept swinging the chair from side to side. Then I felt a hard blow on my back and all the adults jumped on me all at once they pulled me to my feet and holding my arms tight behind my back I was taken to my bed. I was made to lay face down the big fat nurse came to the side of the bed and yanked my jeans down and jabbed a needle in my arse. Pulling my jeans up she said something like "that will keep you quiet" was she right or was she right that was some drug that they gave me. I slept through diner and bedtime; I was awoken by the fat lady walking up and down the dormitory blowing a bloody whistle. What a way to start a day.

I settled down to life here very quickly, I had indeed travelled a long way from my Arthur for I must have slept for hours in Steve's car but I am not silly I knew I could do nothing about it, for here you don't think of your self you just obey.

Every Friday all of us kids took it in turn to see Dr Mead she was the head shrink in fact they all were well I mean they were all psychiatric nurses and Dr Mead was the big knob. I learnt to play a game of my own with them. For if you told them that what they wanted to hear they would leave you alone (believe me it worked) having no room of my own I had no way of talking to my

Lindsay, and to lose both my best friends was unbearable. I found my answer in the large garden for at the far end there was a large big tree. I sat on its trunk and closed my eyes and wiled my Lindsay to come to me. I awoke to find my self in her room. But it was not the same it was Lindsay but not me for my Lindsay was a child I had grown up leaving her behind "WHY" my Lindsay grabbed my hand and pulled me into the corner where we always sat and talked. I could not take my eyes of her. She explained to me talking far beyond her years that she would always remain the age she was when I put her there. In this room for safety she could never grow old or ill or never die I looked at her and said "I put you in here?" she replied "yes" when you could not take no more you put all the good bits of your self and locked them away so they would not be killed. I sat not believing what this child was saying to me and yet deep down I knew it was true.

A question came into my head and I looked straight at her for I needed to know if she was telling the truth. "Are you happy here?" I asked her reply "yes very happy" "but will you always be a kid?" I asked "yes" said Lindsay "always and I will always be here for you until the day we die." Yes we are one we can not live with out each other I thought for a moment and asked her "but don't you ever want to get out of here and live a normal life" I asked my Lindsay looked at me put both her hands either side of my face and said "tonight I will come to you in your dreams and you

will know and understand everything". I opened my eyes and was sitting at the base of the tree.

Twice so far in seven months I have been here I have been restrained and injected, for I have started to fight back and protect myself. Mother's voices had returned frightening at first but I knew I had to over come it somehow. I have also found myself answering her back which made me feel good but only adds fuel to the fire of my insanity. The big fat German lady is a person I hate most every morning she would walk along the line of beds blowing that fucking whistle, so every morning as I woke up my blood would boil.

Timmy Bird a lad who also lives here let me buy his pen knife off him, for fifty pence not bad aye and I would go outside and carve Arthur and my name in a tree, also on the wooden fence post it made me feel that somehow he was here with me. Oh how I miss him, I know I still have my Lindsay and mothers bloody voice but it was Arthur my heart was aching for Dr Mead was a funny woman, it was like she would ask you something then answer it for you. She told me that I had a very big problem with anger and that I must learn to control it better, she asked me if I heard voices in my head "well only if someone was speaking" I answered "no" she said firmly "voices that only I could hear". I looked at her with such a blank expression that she told me to forget it. I walked out of her office knowing that I had to

be a lot more careful, for other wise I would be locked up for ever.

I had no visits; no letters nothing the other kids did but I didn't feel sad for I had my Lindsay. That night as I went to bed I took my opened pen knife with me (I don't know why I swear I had no plan) I placed it under my pillow and soon fell into a peaceful sleep.

I jumped like a frightened animal when the whistle was blown; I hid my head beneath my pillows the sound appeared to be getting nearer. I gripped my penknife so hard my hand was in pain all of a sudden the bedclothes were ripped away from me and the whistle was blown right in my face. I lashed out with my arm and she stumbled backwards (not falling) I jumped out of the bed and stood before her waving my pen knife. "Give me that fucking whistle I screamed at her". "No", no she was trying to say, but I could see the fear in her eyes for now I was the evil one she was the victim. I shouted for all the kids to get out, staff was coming from all directions, I walked nearer to my prey and felt this rush of excitement run through my body (for this I thought must be what it felt like) although it was a pen knife the blade was quite long. Staffs were all around me, Beth was telling me to put the knife down that every thing would be alright, but I knew it would not. Right then, right at that very moment mother said "GO ON STAB THE BITCH" "I cant" I said, mother said "YES YOU CAN NOW DO IT" "I'm not like you" I

shouted then all of a sudden I was pushed to the floor, my knife was pulled from my hand, well you know the rest "injection and sleep". If only it would have been that simple. I awoke to two men pulling me off the bed "walk they said" half dragging me I staggered along the corridor with them. We stopped at the office one man picked a file or something up I was then marched outside and then put in the back of a car. Both men got in either side of me "what's happening, where are you taking me?" but no words were spoken on our five-minute ride. Because I was still drugged I didn't feel no fear, when we stopped I was pulled from the car and dragged up two flights of stairs. They're all I could hear was all these locks and bolts being undone the big steel doors opening. I frog marched in my eyes were all fuzzy couldn't really make much out I heard men talking, I heard one say twelve and a half years old, how could she be mad at such a young age. Do you know it wasn't until the next day I realised he was talking about me? I was taken to a room and made to lie down on a mattress on the floor and then the door was slammed shut and locked behind me. I still didn't feel fear, I just drifted back to sleep without a care in the world (it was the drugs that made me feel like that I had only been given them a few hours earlier which was why I was so out of it).

If I had known that I was now a patient at Grasslands Mental Hospital North Yorkshire in the top security ward with murderers alike, I am sure I

would be very afraid, for I was only twelve and a half years old.

Chapter Eight

My life in the lock up was very tough at first, I was very scared of the men and women there they were like nothing I had ever seen before. I sat on the window ledge and watched them all; in fact I studied them, what made them angry, what made them cry, for the first month I really did nothing else for I had to know my enemy. One person I couldn't make out was a coloured man called Harry, I sat next to him at meal times, the nurses were always asking him things and showing him papers, I surmised that he was F.B.I agent or on a undercover mission for he seemed no madder than I was.

There were just as many staff as there were patients and there were fights breaking out all the time, at first I was scared, but you got used to them. The charge nurse was called Val she was very nice, she explained because of the attack they had no choice but to bring me here. But my social worker Steve King was working on getting me another children's unit somewhere, I understood for I knew that I had done wrong, but with mothers voice fuelling the fire it got out of hand.

On my window sill I sat and lost my self to better things, to me and Arthur walking to school, to Nan giving me a cuddle, to my lady and Auntie Mary, my life was a lot different now and not for the better. There was an old man on the ward he

was called Fred, he was very violent and always being locked in the cells, here too they gave you injections one day as he walked passed me on my window sill he punched me right in the face, I yelled out with pain. I jumped down stood my ground before him, staff was zooming in on us I wanted to hit him back, but he was such an old man staff grabbed Fred marched him off to the cells. I got a pat on the back for not fighting back; my cheek and my eye came up like a balloon.

A few weeks later I was taken down by two nurses to have a brain scan to see if I had one I joked, for I had got close to a lot of the staff, most of them felt sorry for me. Val told me that the whole hospital was talking about me, for a child should not be in a place like this.

Steve King came to see me and he told me that not one of the children's units he had contacted would even consider taking me because of the violence. He had written a letter to the prime minister asking for his help and also, worst of all he had arranged for a Mr Kite (a private tutor) to come for two hours on a Wednesday morning "why?" I asked Steve said "because it is law you must have an education", he gave me some sweets he had bought and told me he would keep in touch.

There are four cells on our ward all the rest were bed rooms, mine was number twelve they had to be kept locked at all times. Otherwise

patients would go in and out of them and pinch things, it was a pain in the arse having to keep asking for my door to be unlocked. It was only the fact that I could spend a lot of time with my Lindsay that kept me going for this was no picnic you had to be on your guard at all times.

Its six months since I had arrived, I have only been in the cells once, and that was for fighting back, Steve has been back a number of times, with no luck, he is going to write to some MPs to see if they can do any good. About ten minutes walk downstairs along lots of corridors there is a hospital shop. I am allowed to go there on my own as long as I am good, it felt so great to get off the ward, I really needed some different views of the world.

It is my birthday today I am thirteen, Val gave me a card and a bag full of sweets, and it meant a lot to me it meant she cared. The rest of the day no one said anything at lunchtime when shifts changed I thought I might get a happy birthday or something from her but no nothing, I sat on my window ledge feeling sorry for myself, when the bell went for tea. I ate my tea in silence with Harry beside me (just what the bloody hell I expected I don't know) as tea was coming to an end, I saw June one of the nurses walking towards me with a cake with candles alight on it the whole ward burst into song I blushed I know I did, but I felt so happy. I blew them all out in two breaths and was told to go and open the door of the big

walk in cupboard near the hatch, I got up and walked to it, the staff gathered round me as I opened the door. My eyes fell upon this red bike with a bow round it. I wheeled it out and gazed at it "but I can't ride" I never learnt don't worry birthday girl, we can soon fix that. Me and my bike taken down stairs to the path on the grounds below my window "I'm not allowed out side I said" "you are now" they replied together and Beth laughed out loud. As long as you behave you can go out each day so come on said Terry get your arse on this bike. With a lot of patients June and Terry (both nurses) jogged up and down with me on the path. I tried to ride a bike at my first children's home but never mastered it completely and yet in half an hour I was riding unaided, wobbly but on my own. Terry let out a yell well done as I rode to the end of the path. I wanted to throw my bike down and hug them both, for I felt so happy. I was allowed out each day to ride my bike round the grounds, it was the first time I realised how big Grasslands was must be hundreds, no thousands of ill people here but also no other children there was a blessing I had my Lindsay to talk to.

There was two locked doors in and out of the ward (ward one) I often wondered why one was never used and unbeknown to me I would soon find out. Val the head charge nurse asked me to go into her office for a chat. I sat on the edge of the chair for it was something I didn't want to hear or I thought it was, Val explained since I

came here I had only been bad once and that since a few months ago on my birthday, I had obeyed the rules and stayed in the grounds so they wanted to take the next step and move me to ward 1A. I sighed I knew my life was too good to be true Val asked me why I wasn't pleased and I told her I liked it here "good" she said and we like you being here but as I did not pose a danger to anyone now and to keep a child in a top security ward was just not RIGHT. Val explained I was only going to be next door I could see them whenever I liked, I only had to ring the buzzer, I explained that I had never been next door, Val said "get your stuff and I will take you". As I packed my bags I still felt sorry, these people, although mad were my friends most of the staff was too. Val came to my room wheeling my bike with her "come on child lets get you out of here" I followed with my heart heavy, Val unlocked the door I followed her through and she put my bike against the wall and relocked the door "we will leave your bike here for now" and with that I followed her down, through the dinning room then left past a lot of doors we stopped at one and Val opened it not with a key just with the handle as I followed her into the room it was the same as my old one, I put my bags on the bed and stood looking miserable "hey kid cheer up its your chance of freedom". Val explained that ward 1A was an open ward as long as I never left the grounds; I was free to come and go, as I liked. I could be out on my bike all day if I wanted, but don't forget she said as she was leaving "you only have to push the buzzer if you

need any of us" she turned and walked out of the room.

Another path of my life had begun, it felt very lonely for there was only one member of staff on at one time, and I didn't know any of them. There was also only six patients including me on the ward, they were old or insane all but one a bloke called Gordon and he was totally out of his tree. He would stand at the end of the long corridor in between the dinning room and the lounge and then suddenly he would run full pelt to the other end, the noise really got to you it was like a herd of animals, and he did it all <u>day every day</u>. I kept my bike in the empty room next door for here nothing had to be kept locked.

For it was very important to me, it was my wheels of freedom, it was while out riding in the grounds one day that I would meet someone he was to play a major part in my life to come (of course neither of us new that). Suddenly my tyre went flat, I stopped and looked at it, sticking out of my tyre was a nail "shit" what now? I said I pulled it out and started to make my way back to the ward 1A over the other side of the road was a works unit, I stood and thought for a moment, "oh well" I said I haven't got anything to lose.

I pushed my bike into this massive workshop place, there was patients making things. A man, (an old man) came from the office looking at me and then the bike "what's up kid" he said I

explained about my bike and he said "if you leave it with me" for I am a bit busy at the moment, and you can come and get it in the morning, it will be fixed. "Thanks mate" I said as he took the bike from me, I will see you in the morning, and I walked back to my ward feeling quite happy with myself.

The next morning, I had a spring in my step; my bike would be fixed and I could enjoy my morning biking around. The man was waiting at the open door, when he saw me, he waved "hi kid come for your wheels" "yes" I said, did you manage to fix it? "See for yourself" he beckoned me to follow him and you will never believe what I saw. Gleaming red bike, new handle bars, saddle, new wheels and the very best thing of all **A BELL**, "wow" I said "that's not my old bike", "correct" he said but it's your new one. I felt like a million dollars "I don't know what to say" no one has ever been this kind to me in my life, thank you mister "well he replied and stop calling me MR and you can call me by my name Les" Les took my bike outside and told me to try it out for size, I rode round and round in his front yard ringing my bell as I went. After a short while Les said he had to get back to work. I thanked him again as I was leaving the yard he shouted to me "you could pop in again if you wanted to" when I was passing. Wow my new bike was great I felt like the queen as I rode around the grounds. This was the best thing that has happened to me in years, maybe my luck was changing.

I think because I was on my own a lot more, mothers voice really got to me sometimes, it was at this time I found out that if I hurt myself, (real pain I mean) then mother left me alone (I know now that this was the start of my self harm) I would look on the ground as I rode my new bike for pieces of glass, or anything sharp really, I hid it in my pocket and when need be cut my arms up, but <u>never</u> below the wrist, for if anyone found out my secret I would be in trouble, but believe you and me it did work. Its funny but I never saw anything. Most kids did silly things so I thought.

Only three months later my nightmares came true, and again I was a victim, nothing different happened that day, and I went to bed as normal and slept well, that was until I woke up terrified, a hand over my mouth I struggled to breath, "lay still and you wont get hurt" a mans voice said, I knew what was going to happen, my pyjama bottoms were pulled down and this enormous man lay on top of me, he moved his hand away from my mouth and moved to guide his penis into me, at this point I started to scream out but his hand slapped back over my mouth, " just enjoy it baby" he whispered as he was jerking up and down, finally he came and he relaxed his hand from my mouth, the smell of him was like nothing on this earth. He got off me and slowly he in front of me he pulled his trousers back up, then without a word he walked out of my room and closed the door, I pulled my pyjama trousers up and the covers and lied there a totally broken

child, all I had for comfort was my teddy from my Nan's. I decided that night I didn't want to live anymore, nothing was worth the pain I had to go through, this time I would die for sure, I would make a good job of it. I laid all night, no Lindsay, no Arthur and no mother, "alone".

Next morning without even washing I got my small amount of money and wheeled my bike down the corridor for the very last time. I left the grounds for search for shops, I went into a shop and bought one hundred aspirins and a bottle of cheap lemonade and then I rode back to the hospital, to my favourite spot by the big tree, next to some waste land, and one by one I swallowed all the pills. I sat feeling really sick, and wanted to die, there was no way I was going to fail or chicken out, my head started to go all funny and I can't remember saying out loud something like " goodbye Arthur, I love you".

I opened my eyes, everything was a daze, I tried to focus, I was in heaven, all these years I didn't believe in it, but it was the truth, or was it "No" I yelled "No" I don't want to live, let me die, I sat up there was tubes everywhere I grabbed at them yanking them out there were nurses trying to hold me down, but I was hysterical, I herd the nurse shouting for help, then nothing I had been knocked out I think by injection, for when I awoke, Val was sitting in a chair next to me she looked very concerned "why?" she asked, but I just looked straight through her. I had no words for

anyone. I had nearly died; a workman had found me near to death. I had been asleep for over a week, I had, bags upon bags of fluid and blood, I was so very lucky to be alive that's what they said. Staff from ward 1 came to see me, so many of them but they all asked the same question "why?" I don't know if I was just to broken hearted, or scared, or embarrassed to tell them what had happened, but like always I remained silent. When at last I was discharged from hospital I was taken back to ward 1, where all my things had been moved back to, for this I was most grateful. To be with patients and staff I knew easier.

My bike was taken away from me, not that I had the energy or the heart for it. The nurses were very kind to me and the weeks that followed, but my spirit had gone, I cursed God for not taking me, for how, could he make his children suffer so much.

A man came a few weeks later to set some schoolwork. I just sat and stared at him, I think he left with his tail between his legs. I suppose it must be at least six weeks later when Val my favourite nurse was sitting talking to me, (like she often did) when suddenly I burst out crying, with Val's arms gently holding me, I told her about the rape, she rocked me back and fourth telling me everything would be alright, the relief I felt was enormous, she gave a pill and laid me down to sleep on my bed telling she would not leave.

I awoke during the night; I left my room in search for my window sill. The next day, two police officers came on to the ward; I was soon summoned to the office. The police woman told me I had to make a statement of what had happened and with a male nurse, and a man and lady police officer, I had to recall everything that happened that night, I felt that they thought it was my fault, they had asked had I led him on, I was just so flabbergasted, I was a thirteen and a half year old mental patient, what did they think I had done.

For the next three months no one said a word about it, until one day Val sat beside me on the window sill and quietly told me "that my rapist had been stripped of being a nurse for life and he was an in-patient in another mental hospital" and that he would remain there for a long time. Finally justice had been done, not that I would ever forget what he had done for me, but it would be easier to live with, for that's just what I had to do, I had been through so much, but I knew I had to reach adult hood, for then only then I can find my beloved brother. I continued to serve my days with faith in my heart.

One day a few weeks later, Steve King came out of the blue, he was very excited and told me to wait for him, he just had to go to the office first. When he came out he came rushing over to me saying, "Pack your bags Lindsay your getting out" "what, where?" "an adolescence unit in

Cambridge has accepted you. We are to leave immediately." "But I can't" I told him, I have to say goodbye to my friends, Steve told me I had thirty minutes and then we had to go. A nurse came and helped me pack my bags after, I walked around the ward saying goodbye to all my fellow patients, but my best friend was not on duty today, Terry said he would tell Val I said goodbye. "My bike" I said, I have got to take my bike, Steve didn't like it, but he could also see I meant what I said, while he was getting my things loaded up, I ran around to the workshop, I told Les everything that had happened and he seemed sad, I looked straight into his eyes and told him I would miss him, and that he was a very good friend. He wrote down as much of the address that I knew and told me he would try and visit. I hugged him, like I had never dared to do to any other male I knew, and felt a warmth from him that was like nothing I had ever felt before, as I turned and walked away, I had the feeling we would see each other again. Steve was waiting by his car, pacing up and down. Come on he said, "I would have thought that you couldn't have waited to get out of this place".

As I always did, I stood and looked up at the windows of my ward, then climbed into the car to start yet another part of my life.

Chapter Nine

I found out on our journey a lot of things I didn't know, Steve told me that over a hundred letters had been wrote to the M.P`s, health authorities, even parliament tried to get me (a minor) out of Grasslands Mental hospital, he also told me that my name was known up and down the country by anyone that could help. I sat dumb struck, but why? I asked, because it was against the law for you to be there he said. "So why was I put in there?" I asked, because you attacked a member of staff, you was classed as dangerous, you was only supposed to be there for a few days at the most, I could not think of anything else to say, so he drove in silence, both deep in our own thoughts. A while later I was the first to break silence, "how far is Cambridge away from Littleton" I asked, "I'm not sure exactly, but around seventy miles or so, too far for you to walk home he laughed". I smiled, but not at him, for I was thinking I was getting nearer to Arthur, and that was good for me. Steve explained that Highlands Adolescence unit was in the grounds of a disused hospital, there was woods all around, and the manager is called Mrs Game she had worked with disturbed children, for many years. The unit is run like a family home, and like every where else I had lived all the staff were nurses, it housed only twelve children at a time it was a very "one to one unit" he also said how lucky I was to get a place there.

We turned off and went down a really long lane, Steve pointed to his right and told me that was the disused hospital, he turned left and pulled up against this great big bloody house. The first thing I saw was bike racks so I hopped out of the car he heaved my bike out of the boot, and put it in the rack, there was quite a few in there.

Steve introduced me to Mrs Game. She was coloured, she took my bags and lead me up a flight of stairs, there was rooms every where, she walked into one, and placed my bags on the first bed you came too, (there was three beds in the room) and a lot of furniture, it was a large room, Mrs Game explained that there was four bedrooms all the same, three children in each, and two big bathrooms upstairs and two single toilets down stairs, she told me to follow her down and she would show me the rest of the house. For that's what it was, not a unit or hospital. I asked where the other children were, she replied "well at school where else? Of course you have not been for a long time, but here you will go, for it is the law that every child should have an education". She had a smile on her face while she was saying that, I knew I would like this woman.

I sat in the kitchen, flanked either side by Steve and Mrs Game, when all of a sudden I could hear children's voices, it sounded really strange, for two years I had not even seen another kid, and as the noise got louder, I felt a little afraid. As the back door was flung open in came an array of

kids, all sizes and colours. Mrs Game stood up and asked them to remain in the kitchen for a minute so she could introduce the new kid (me) one by one they said their names and I replied "hello" they all looked normal. One lad with blonde hair caught my eye for I think I could see something in his eyes that were in mine. Mrs Game told the children that they could go, but could Sarah and Jane remain for a few minutes. When they had all filed out Mrs Game asked the two girls, if they could take me under their wings for a few days to show me the ropes, they both agreed quite willingly, I said my good byes to Steve, and was taken upstairs to unpack, Sarah and Jane laid on their beds asking questions while I unpacked my stuff. I told them as little as possible, for it was the best way. I asked them what they thought of Mrs Game, and they both replied she is fine, OK.

Life settled down very quickly for me at Highlands it was indeed a house, not a unit. There was rota in the kitchen for every day, we all had a job to do, you would do it for a week then the rota would change and you had a different one for the following week and so on. I fell in love with the woods around us straight away; they gave me a sense of belonging and safety, for in them you couldn't see the **SKY**, and evil that was always lurking around. I made friends with most of the other kids, but the blonde haired one named Josh, I was very drawn too, Sarah told me, not to go near him, that he was as mad as a hatter, but the

134

first time I saw him, I saw some of me in him. He was indeed very odd, he was also by all accounts quite violent but this certainly didn't worry me, for after two years in a top security ward I could handle myself quite nicely. I don't know if Josh could see himself in me also, but within days we had become friends. The rules were very flexible and gave us a lot of our time to ourselves. We were allowed to ride around the grounds, or play in the woods or to explore the outside grounds of the disused hospital, there was always something to do, but if you wanted to go into town or buy things like that then you had to get a pass from Mrs Game, we also was given one pound pocket money each week from the government.

School was a piece of cake. Mrs Jones was the teacher. She was a complete walk over. I told her that had not attended school since I was eleven. (Which was not a lie). So until she could get my records from Meadow View Secondary. I could just write stories and do work from puzzle books. School was a real joke not only for me but all of us, except one. Annabel she was a real snob, she was from a well to do family. She even owned two horses and felt she was above all of us, no one really liked her. But we all had to put up with her. Her clothes, the way she walked, even the way she talked was all above any of us. And she was always making it clear, that unlike us she should not be here. It was all a big mistake, and her daddy was getting it sorted out. She had this small bottle of stuff. What it was I don't know and

she spent all day putting it up her nostril and sniffing, it made me feel really sick, (it was not medicine just something you could buy over the counter).

As Josh and me were digging out a den in the woods, I was telling him how pissed off I was with Annabel, I told him I had a plan to make her look stupid. He told me to go for it. We had worked for two days digging; it was nice being with someone my own age. I liked Josh he was alright. We never talked about our lives. We had a rule, that anything that had happened before we met was <u>spent</u>, never to be unearthed; that was just fine by me, I think that's why we got on so well, for we knew that neither one of us would want answers to questions we didn't want to say.

After tea that evening I lay on the settee in the TV room and felt very lucky, I had not realised how much I had missed other children. The worst bit about Highlands was the weekly visits of our friendly psychiatrist Dr Woodcock; he was a real prat. He told me on our first meeting that I had a split personality, and that I was quite badly disturbed, and with his help and Highlands I could improve myself quite substantially "stupid bastard" I said to myself as I left the office, who the fuck does he think he is. In fact I remained in a bad mood for the rest of the day.

I lay in my bed, thinking what that stupid doctor had said and decided; I had to find out what

he meant. I decided to ask Mrs Game in the morning.

I awoke "screaming". I sat in the dark with John the night nurse beside me. I was trembling with fear. I was soaked with sweat, for mother had stabbed ME <u>not the pillow</u>, and she stood above me laughing, my nightmares are becoming a lot more often now, but as always I kept what they were about to myself. Sarah and Jane my room mates learned not to ask. For they would get a mouthful back, for I had become one of the top ranking kids in the place by then, I was almost one to be feared, for I think I gave off a scent, that I was an alpha female. Looking back it was a good thing, because no one got too close, well except Josh. In the morning I asked as planned what split personality was, and Mrs Game, explained that's its meaning were two minds in one body. I sat looking straight through her, was that what I was, she was still talking but heard no more of her words. Over and over I kept saying her words, two minds in one, two minds in one, I left the kitchen and said, "I was going for a walk, for in the woods I knew I could think by myself. All day I moved around the woods my mind totally screwed up I just could not think in a straight line if you know what I mean, for I had always been told, I was disturbed and that had never bothered me until now. I would not go home tonight. I would stay in the den in the woods. And be with my Lindsay that's if my mind would let me. Our den was right in the heart of the woods from there you could not

see Highlands to the left and the lane and hospital to the right. I had never spent the night out before and certainly not in woodlands. But none of that came to my head, I was not cold because I was in our den, I had no wind on me, I sat propped up against the balk wall, and tried to let my mind go, but Mrs Games words kept going on and on. I hit my head several times against the sidewall, and they started to fade, but when I stopped they returned "I knew what I had to do" I crawled out and stood up, walked to the nearer tree and started pounding my head against its trunk, again, and again, I felt no pain for I never did, I stopped for I felt water running down my face, I stood listening for any voices but still I could hear her. I turned my body around and started pounding the back of my head the next thing I had knew I had fell to the ground, I remember the smell of the earth and the leafs against my face. Crawling back into our den I tasted blood in my mouth I felt my hair it was wet through and so was my face, but not with water as I had thought but with blood. I lay in our den and went to be with my Lindsay. Just the sight of her made me feel better, I slowly told her what had happened that day, her answer (what made perfect sense) was that I know what and who I am, and as long as I knew it didn't matter what anyone else thought. I knew Lindsay would have the answer I told her about mother in my dreams and all she said was that all they were were dreams. Of course again she was right it seemed odd, for my Lindsay had a brain of some one a lot older than her eight or nine years. I think

I must have fell for light was pouring in the entrance to our den, I crawled out and stood up and stretched, oh God my head hurts. My hair is all matted on my head, and slowly the memories come back of the night before. I walked slowly home stumbling as I went.

As I entered the kitchen Mrs Game was drinking a cup of something, she jumped up and came over to me, saying where had I been what had happened to my head, did I know that the police was out looking for me all night. I just stood there. She grabbed my face in her hands and asked. "What the hell had happened to me"? I replied. "I fell over and knocked my head on a tree". She turned me around and was touching my head all over. I did not like this I pulled away telling her to leave me alone, I think she realised this so she backed away from me. I walked upstairs and grabbed some clean clothes and went to have a shower. My head was full of lumps and cuts, but now it was washed and when it had dried no one would notice, but my face was a different kettle of fish, I would work that one out as I went along.

As I went down to breakfast with everyone else Josh gave me a nod and a look to say glad you are all right. The others knew not to say anything after breakfast I was told to wait in my bedroom until Dr Woodcock arrived "But school" I said but the look was enough to tell me not to argue. I lay on my bed waiting to see what my punishment would be. A lady nurse I forgot her

name came into my room. "Letter for you" she said and placed it on the bottom of my bed. I picked it up, it had my name on the front but I had never had a letter in the whole of my life I lay looking at it, I undone it with great care as not to damage the envelope at all. The letter was from Les Barnes at Grasslands Metal Hospital, he said "it took him all these weeks to find out where I had gone" it carried on about my bike and asking how the other kids was. And was I going to school. And how he missed me biking around his yard. He had also put in his letter a few pieces of paper and an envelope with his name and address on it, and a stamp on it, so as he says in his letter if I feel like writing back I can. He also explained that his wife Pat would like to meet me and the letter carried on about Grasslands and things, and at the end it said "be good kid, be thinking of you, write back if you can bye for now Les".

It was a nice letter except the bit about Pat. For it was Les that was my friend not her, I opened the other one and indeed there was paper folded up in it, all I had to do was to put the words in.

I was summoned to the office by Mrs Game, Dr Woodcock was behind his desk "sit down" he said I sat down for I knew I just had to go it alone and agreed with them. That's always seemed to work for me. He gave me a lecture about wasting police time. And that they were responsible for me and my well being and that I

had been given a chance in life being allowed to come to Highlands, he carried on and on and then he stood up and walked around the side of the table. He stretched his arms out to touch me; I jumped out of my chair and backed myself into a corner. I put my hands up to my face to protect my self. Dr Woodcock jumped but then he had realised what he had done, Mrs Game stood up and was telling me that it was ok. I saw Woodcock go back to the other side of the table, and then took my chance and opened the door and legged it back to my bedroom and I slammed the door and slid down onto my bum and cried. Dr Woodcock was a jumped up mind bending psycho, but just the thought of a man touching me was enough to make me run like a scared rabbit. About an hour later Mrs Game came in and said that Dr Woodcock had asked her to apologise for him, and that it very thoughtless of him, I said nothing I just sat there. She also said "that a female doctor was coming to look at my head". "I told her that there was no need" but she didn't agree and anyway she said it was policy. As to her word later a lady G.P came to my room and went all over my head, eyes, face, asking if I had an headache, or double vision, or a ringing in my ears. For she was very good. I told her I did have a headache. And with that she sat on my bed. "I bet you have" she knew not to bother to ask how I had got this way. She wrote out a note or something and said. "She would give something" and that I was to get into bed and remain there for the next two days I started to argue but knew

there was no point, so when she left I got my night clothes and quite gratefully climbed into bed. Sleep soon took hold of me, and the dreams stayed away, for that I was most grateful.

I did send a letter back to Les about a week later "why?" well I remember the cuddle he gave me when I was parting. It was unlike any I had ever got from a male before, I felt I needed a friend, and I knew he was that, and if I didn't like Pat I knew that I had not lost nothing.

Josh knew that I was in our den the night I was missing, we were more alike than I was comfortable with, but I also liked the excitement that together we had, and I was scared of nothing, the same as him. I suppose looking back, that neither of us had much to lose. In the time we were friends there was never anything else between us, for both of us had been hurt beyond repair.

Yesterday afternoon I was lying on the settee trying not to listen to mother. When suddenly I could not take anymore and shouted at her to leave me alone, Sarah was in the room and burst out laughing, I jumped up went over to her and bashed her as hard as I could straight in the face. As I turned Mrs Rose (a nurse) was standing in the doorway, she shouted at me to get upstairs and in my room. Sarah was balling her eyes out. I heard a car come and go but I didn't bother to look out of my window to see who it was for later I

would find out myself. Mrs Game came in same as usual what had I done, I told her that Sarah was taking the mickey out of me and she said she found it very hard to believe. Anyway I stuck to my story and she left, saying that Sarah had been taken to a hospital to be checked out, I laughed but stopped almost immediately at the look on Mrs Game's face it felt just lately I was always in trouble. I had to learn not to answer mother back. I made a pact with myself that I would go back to cutting myself to control her voice.

Sarah came back that evening with a white plaster thing straight across the brow of her nose, I had broken it "shit now I would be in trouble" but I didn't care, it was her own fault anyway it was her word against mine.

I started to quite enjoy school, Mrs James was not bad really, I started to enjoy writing stories, and sometimes I would put a bit of myself into them. One day she asked me to write about feelings. Well I knew a lot about them. So that essay not too difficult. May be I went too far. For Mrs James was pleased in fact so pleased she wanted to show it to Dr Woodcock. In a panic I grabbed my paper and ran out of class I was tearing it up into little pieces as I was going, I had made a "big mistake" I must never let anyone into my head, from now, I must be on guard at all times. I carried on running all the way to the den. Once inside I dug bottle end out of the dirt and began taking my punishment I was a coward. I

scarred my body over and over again, just for mother.

Les sent me another letter. Again he enclosed paper and envelope for me to write back. Also he sent a photo of him and pat his wife, they looked very nice together and very happy, he was so pleased I had wrote back and asked if I would like him and pat to visit me one weekend, he said to let him know, when I wrote back. As I read I had a warm feeling come over me, I don't know if it was because he was a nurse and that's why I thought he understood me more.

Shit or bust, I thought, I replied I would love to see them, but I also said that I hadn't been very good so I didn't know if Mrs Game would allow it. I waited eagerly for a reply, for Les had always been very kind to me, and what with everything that was going on at the moment I could do with a bit of friendship. I was really lucky, for five days later one Thursday afternoon after school. Mrs Game told me that a Mr Les Barnes had been on the phone to her. He explained who he was and had requested a visit for Saturday afternoon. I looked right into her eyes. Just waiting to hear the words yes or no. My luck was really in they had agreed. "Yes". I yelled and started to dance around my bedroom. Mrs Game stood at the door watching me flabbergasted. As she had never really seen me happy before, when I had calmed down she asked me to sit on the bed and explain why these people got a reaction from me. I told

her the story of my bike and how. Without wanting anything from me. He had transformed my bike into something of a dream to ride. I also told her about my visits to his yard. And how he was a charge nurse and had been for thirty years, how he was very old, but yet understood me, like no other really and last of all, about my good bye cuddle. I had tears in my eyes and a frog in my throat when I was telling her. And gently she put her arm around me. And talked softly to me saying I had, had such a hard life, and it must have been hell living at the mental hospital, and if this Les Barnes and his wife made my happy as they obviously did, then she would do everything to back their visits. I allowed myself to be cuddled and must admit it felt good.

I was walking up and down in front of the house my stomach was really nervous, they were coming at two PM, every five minutes or so I ran into see what time the kitchen clock said. That was the longest forty minutes of my life. At last Les's car pulled up and stopped outside of the house, I ran over to open his door also trying to get a look at Pat at the same time. I opened his door and Les got out he took me in his arms and cuddled me then swung me around. "Good kid I've missed you" he said. Come and meet the wife Les opened the door and out came a nice quiet lady. Fancy hair, nice clothes, with a large smile on her face. She took my hand and said "it a pleasure to meet you Lindsay I have heard so much about you, I hope we too can become friends" I took her

hand then I asked if they would like to come in, as we headed for the kitchen Door. I felt that I would know these people for a very long time to come. Les talked to Mrs Game, and I was left with Pat, I did feel a little bit weird, but I guessed she did as well. She asked about school and the other children, just general things but it made me feel at ease more with her. In the corner of the kitchen was a stack of games she asked if I liked them. I admitted I had not played any of them before Les came back in with Mrs Game. "Oh kid there's something for you in the boot of the car, run and get it". With that he threw a bunch of keys at me, "black one" he said I ran out of the door as fast as my legs could carry me, for I was not accustomed to getting presents. In the boot was a dustbin liner full of stuff. I lifted it out and locked the boot and returned the keys to Les in the kitchen. I put the bag on the table and started to go through it. There were sweets galore, a puncher repair kit, writing paper and envelopes and stamps. Felt tip pens and colouring pencils, colouring book, sketch pad, a packet of five white girls socks and like a see-through plastic case for all my drawing stuff. Oh and a ruler and rubber set, I kissed Les and thanked Pat very much they were both too kind, I took my bag of goodies up to my room for safe keeping.

I made Les and Pat a cup of tea and we sat in the TV room talking, Les said as long as I behave myself that Mrs Game could se no reason why we could not make this a regular thing. Pat

said she wanted to ask me something but did not want me to take it the wrong way. I told her to just ask. "Well your clothes" she said "look a bit worn out and old. I was wondering if you would let us get you some new ones". My reply was. "I do get a clothing grant of thirty pounds a year. But last year I had to spend it all on clothes and shoes. Why should you waste all your money on clothes for me?" "Well that's easy" said Les "it's because we both like you and care a lot about you" is that not a good enough reason? I replied with sorrow in my heart "I have nothing to give back in return" Les said "but Lindsay but of course you do, you give us your friendship, for that is all we ask". Then said Les "next visit we go shopping." I sat and looked at these two people and asked myself why had they picked me out of the normal kids in the world why me? Did friends do all that sort of stuff for each other, I didn't think so. I got mad at myself for questioning myself over a good thing; I suppose it was because I had never had it before. When it was time for them to leave I felt very sad, in fact I didn't think they were out of the lane for I was missing them and longing for the next Saturday to come. Mrs Game had agreed to us going out on our outing, as long as I was good. I went and very neatly put all my things in a folder then in my cupboard I put my socks in my knickers drawer. Do you know it was very hard for me to like anyone? And here I was having to control my every thought and behave to get another visit from them but most well nearly, all the time shit just

happened, it was not planned before hand, so it was going to be a very hard week.

Josh and I had for a long time tried to think of a way of getting the posh girl Annabel back. For being so la de da, I had thought of a way, I asked Josh to come outside to have a look at my bike for me (because Mrs Game had eyes everywhere, and because I had to be good). I told him all about my plan and he fell about laughing at my idea so together we decided tonight. We would do it. During that evening I had only had to look at Josh and laughed, it was nice for both of us to feel happy. About an hour or so. After lights out I lay in my bed which faced the door. And waited for my plan to start. Josh appeared in the darkness in my doorway and waved for me to join him. In a flash I was out of bed and beside him, he passed me the bottle and I quickly went into the toilets, it took me ages to do my bit, eventually I completed my task. And crept to Josh's door way and gave him the bottle. With a ten foot wide smile on his face, I retired to my bed for the night, for only the morning would tell if the plan had worked.

I think Josh and me were the first down for breakfast, for we both felt like naughty little school kids, but we were made to wait until nearly school time to see our plan start to work. Josh and me nearly fell out of the kitchen doors on our way to school, for I think we nearly wet ourselves with laughter but Josh said "we must control our laughter because we will give our game away" and

of course he was right. That day was a good day for one and all. I couldn't remember when I had so much fun; Josh was a good lad to be with. Neither of us were cowards, we both didn't have much to lose, so really nothing was out of bounds. Maybe an older and wiser person could see that together we were a bomb waiting to explode.

Dr Woodcock told me I looked happier, I think I even gave him a smile he also said "I was to start taking some medication just to see if it made me not feel so confused and messed up". I started to object when he butted in and said "it will only be trial for a short while". I explained to him that at hospital I had to take pills and they just made me feel sleepy all the time, he looked through my notes and assured me that it was just for mood swings and had no side effects, he also added that if I wanted trips and visits I had to give a little too. I knew what he was saying, and I agreed to take the pills morning and night. As I walked out of his office I said "bastard" under my breath, in this life you never get anything for nothing I thought to myself as I went to find Josh.

He was sat in the TV room in a chair with his knees up chuckling to himself while Sarah and Annabel sat talking, in her hand was the bottle of nostril cleaner, I walked over and told Josh to come outside with me, as we walked out Josh was trying to hold back the floods of tears, once outside he burst into laughter, I tried to calm him down for I needed to talk to him, but it was harder

than I thought for every time he stopped laughing and I started telling him about Dr Woodcock he would just burst into laughter again. I just had enough; I turned and walked away from him into the woods on my own. A few minutes later Josh caught up with me saying how sorry he was, I started to tell him on our walk to the den about the pills that Woodcock had said I must take. He agreed that he was a bastard, and told me to flush them down the pan he said "that's what he does with his" I looked at him and said," I didn't know you took pills". He just grinned and said, "I don't". With a smile on his face Josh told me that Annabel had came into the kitchen this morning and threw her bottle away. Josh asked her why she had done that and she quite simply said, "it was empty" with that we both burst out laughing, we laughed so much we felt sick, so little miss Annabel likes sniffing piss. Josh said "oh yes don't you know posh people do it all the time".

Saturday twelve o'clock on the dot Les and Pat drove up to the house, Les got out and came into see Janice (new day nurse) to say we was off to town she said "have a good time" "don't worry" said Les "we will". The car was very hot inside I asked Les how far away his house was and he replied "about an hour or so". I was shocked that they came so far just to see me; it felt good being with Les and Pat for I could feel the love they had for each other. I asked them if I could ask them some stuff and Les said, "I could ask whatever I wanted" my first question was "why didn't they

have any kids of their own". Pat turned and looked at me and answered "I cannot have children, I had to have something called a hysterectomy when I was just twenty two" which means I can not bare any children. I looked into her face and could see the pain my question had caused her "I'm sorry Pat I did not mean to hurt you" "oh it's ok Lindsay you didn't know" but I knew her words were a lie. "Next question" Les said but I had no more to ask now I knew what I wanted to know. We parked in the multi story car park on level six. As we waited for the lift, I suddenly had the urge for a cuddle and without thinking I grabbed Pat tight and cuddled her with the feelings I never knew I had. As we walked around the shops I held Pat and Les's hand. I felt like a million dollars, I was so proud of them both and hoped everyone would think I was their kid just out on a shopping trip. They both bought me masses of clothes, jeans, trousers, tops, jumpers, trainers, and underwear. Pat asked me what size bra I was and she was very surprised, when I whispered that I didn't have one. With that she told Les to go and get us a seat in the burger bar and that we would be along soon. He took all the bags and left us in the department store Pat asked if I would let her measure me in the changing rooms so as we could get the right size bra. Feeling a bit embarrassed I agreed. We went into a cubicle and I removed my jumper. I went to take off my tee shirt when Pat said there was no need. She could measure over the top. I must admit I was very grateful. She was a very gentle lady. She asked if

I wanted her to pick one and bring it in. I replied "yes please I am new at this". A few minutes later Pat returned with two bras a black one and a beautiful laced white one she said "it would be best if I tried one to check" and she left me alone. I looked into the mirror and saw not a mad little brat. But a young lady Pat was just as nice as Les, for on this day they made me feel like someone very special, when in fact it was them that was the special ones for how they could see good in me I didn't know.

My nightmares continued much to Sarah's and Jane's disgust. Sarah even asked to be moved to another room, my nights were becoming worse than my days. I took the pills Dr Woodcock had given me; they didn't do anything as far as I could tell. But some things had started to happen, which was all down to me, we were allowed to ride or walk to the local shops to spend our pocket money. One day Josh and I went, and well to cut a long story short he taught me to shop lift. I must say he didn't make me I knew what I was doing but it gave me a buzz to come out of shops with stuff I didn't pay for. There were four shops in a row we used, flower shop, bakers, post office and news agents it was the latter one which was my favourite. I was not proud of what I was doing, for I knew it was wrong, but it didn't stop me. Getting caught and the shopkeeper calling the police was the only way I was to learn. Mrs Game was disgusted with me, but no more than myself. I was not made to do it I did it to get a buzz and for that I

was to pay. Two months later I stood in a juvenile court and received a fine of ten pounds, and I knew I deserved it and far more, I was disgusted at myself, but most of all I had let Les and Pat down.

Chapter Ten

I have been at Highlands Adolescence unit for a little over a year, in my time here I have been in a lot of trouble, but having my woods was the best part of it all. Do you know I knew them like the back of my hand, even in the dark I could run through them with no fear of getting hurt? Because you see no sky (well not a mass) mother's powers are not so strong. It was like my Garden of Eden.

My shame over the shop lifting took a heavy toll on me; I had to punish myself a great deal for it was truly an evil thing to do. Mothers voice was making me suffer for it as well I had cut my arms to pieces, but that was not enough I must suffer more, so as not to disobey mother. I knew what I had to do but I didn't give in easily, for the woods were a part of me. But as instructed I set off on my punishment, I had matches that I had stolen, and I went to the far side of the woods where I gathered lots of twigs and leaves. Then I set light to my Garden of Eden. I stood and watched as the fire grew very quickly, mother was laughing louder and louder, I turned and ran, clutching my head in both hands for my pain was unbearable. I was lucky for as I ran through the house to my bedroom no one was around. "What the HELL had I done" I had destroyed a piece and sanctuary. I for once did not know what to do. Soon I heard the sound of fire engines and hope they could soon put it out, my heart was pumping

like mad as I lay, remembering what I had done. Mother was pleased and I knew that she would leave me in peace for a while.

It was three days until I could sneak out to see what mother made me do. A large area had been burnt to the ground; she was pleased with her handy work. I began to think if there was anything I could do to make amends, for although it was mothers' doing it was by my hand.

Dr Woodcock and Mrs Game had done like a rota on whether or not I could see Les and Pat. In two weeks time I was going on an overnight stay at their home, I was looking forward to it. I had begun to look at Les and Pat as more than friends; I had real feelings for them and knew they felt the same for me. Les wrote about twice a week pages full of news from Grasslands and a message from my friend Val to keep my chin up and work hard at school. I looked forward to my letters they had become a bit of sanity. Josh was not well he had voices but lots of them. I knew how hard it was with just having mothers. So I can only imagine what my friend had to cope with, like me he had good days and bad days but he seemed to have a lot more bad days lately. I was worried about him, and so I found out later I had good reason to be. He was off school so I never saw him much during the days and two days later we got back from school the house was in an up roar. Woodcock was here Mrs Game and a police car out front I knew at once it was Josh. We was

all made to go into the TV room and Janice the nurse on duty stood by the door making sure we stayed put. We could hear Josh screaming and shouting. We heard people shouting back. I could hear the fear in his voice. I begged Janice to let me go up and talk to him. I told her we were best friends. That he would listen to me, then we heard a crash and saw the body falling past the window to the ground the kids were going hysterical, I stood for I knew that was my friends body was laying on the front lawn for all to see. In a flat second there were people all around him, and in the longest five minutes of our lives we heard and saw the ambulance take our friend away. All us kids was in shock and more staff were called in for the night duty, for the kids to talk to. I lay on my bed and remained silent, for although he was my best friend I had ever had I knew what Josh went through each day, just to survive. He had often talked about how much easier it would be just to end it all. I lay all night going over all my time with Josh. And felt lucky to have known him, for although we had not been told he had died (he had broken his neck) I knew he had for I could not feel him, we were told the next day that Josh was very ill, also that none of it was anyone's fault, and for us all to remember Josh as he was when he was well.

I felt like shouting and screaming saying that they didn't even know the real Josh, but by then I like most was in a state of shock. All leave was cancelled, because the nurses came in from

God knows where to counsel all the kids, I with a few other kids still could not talk about it.

We were not allowed to go to his funeral because Josh's mum lived a long way away so he was buried up near his real home. It took weeks for the home to get back to normal again kids would be eating and suddenly burst into tears the worst thing for me and most was seeing the body go past the window and the sound it made hitting the ground. I kept trying to tell myself that at last he would be at peace and be one again.

Three weeks after Josh's death I was still numb I had not been able to really cry, (that's why Mrs Game did what she did). I was in the TV room when in walked Les and Pat, I ran into their open arms and wept like a baby, Pat was crying too they had gentle words and open arms for me. Pat took me upstairs and packed my nightclothes and other clothes and put my coat on me and led me gently downstairs and out to their car. Pat sat cuddling me in the rear of the car as Les were saying words of comfort from the front. It was dark and cold, but being with them made life seem not so bad. We drove for a long time, and then we pulled into the driveway of this small house. Pat got out and helped me out and together the three of us what was to become my new home. (But not quite that easy). It was small but very nice and homely, they showed me all the rooms and where I would be sleeping, but my eyes were very sore from all the crying I had done. Les asked me if I

knew why Josh had done it so I explained how Josh's life was "poor kid" Pat said "it must be hard on you as well, what with the voices". Well you could have knocked me down with a feather, as I sat opened mouth lost for words, Les realised what Pat had said and started telling me that everyone had a hang up, and that mine was no worse than the next person's. I don't really know what I was thinking relief I suppose but no one ever knew about mother before, or so I thought. But as Les explained nurses was trained to look for problems like these, I asked him who told him and in a matter of a fact way he noticed it the first few times I had bike around his yard. He told me to sit on his lap he wanted to explain something to me, I had never feared Les at all, and so I did as he asked with his arms around me and Pat beside us he told me that no matter what was wrong with me that him and Pat loved me very much and if I felt the same way about them as they thought I did, he would apply to foster me and if successful I would become their daughter. I burst out crying and the three of us were hugging and crying together. After a few minutes Les said to me "I take it it is a yes then" "YES PLEASE" I shouted for the world to hear we cuddled again and as we parted my face changed "but there was so much you don't know about me I have done some bad things". Pat took my face in her hands and looking straight at my eyes she said "love can overcome any hurdles put in it's path" then she kissed me on the lips she told me she would be honoured to have me in their family. My whole life changed that

night, for here are two people who didn't care how mad I was, they just loved me. Les said I didn't have to return until six pm Sunday so that would give us all the time in the world to say what we wanted to. One thing that they would ask of me is that I never lied to them. I gave them both my words on the spot. I slept well in my bed in my tiny new room for I had never been so happy. Before I went to sleep that night I said good bye to my very best friend and hoped he was one again.

Laying in bed in the morning I kept thinking about what Les had said that he noticed I had voices right at the start, if he knew others must, but no one had ever asked about them for it had been my secret since the age of eleven and I was not sure that if Les and Pat knew about mother and the things I did for her, they would still love me. I mean how could I tell them about the fires, cutting myself up I mean it all made sense to me but I was to blame for doing them I was sure they wouldn't understand. I had known them now for a year and a half they never knew much bad about me (the shop lifting they knew) for I was never caught for the fire. My mind was so mixed up, I loved them I think well I sure did care about them more than anybody else (except Arthur) but to me love was a very unexplained word, for if it was love I felt for my brother, then its not love I feel for the Barnes. I decided I had to try and explain this to them, I dressed and went downstairs, they were both in the kitchen reading news papers at the table I sat and tried to explain my worries. They so

understood and Les seemed to get just what I was trying to say. I told them about my brother and how close we were, but nothing at all about mother or William for if they knew about them they most certainly not want me. On and off all day long we talked, at one stage Les said "that if I wanted we just could remain as we are". I saw the hurt in both their eyes after he suggested it, I assured them both that I wanted what they did but they had to understand I was no normal kid. I asked them why they had never adopted or fostered before, and they said it was just the hand they had been dealt, and so they flung themselves into their works. It was only when I came into their lives, that having a kid to care for, and love was a very precious gift, and one they had secretly both wanted all their married life. Les asked when my birthday was I replied "eighth of the ninth sixty two" Les said "hell that's only a few weeks away, and you will be of legal age anyway, this is going to easier than I thought". Pat asked what present I would like from them I replied "I don't know and that I didn't even realise it was my birthday soon". We sat in silence all deep in our thoughts. Les spoke first saying first thing Sunday morning he would set the ball rolling, and I would soon be calling his home my home as well. I looked at him and without realising I said "not until I am seventeen not sixteen" Les looked at me "what do you mean" he asked I replied calmly that I was on a care order until I was seventeen that hurt Les and I regretted saying it but it was the truth. On

our journey back to Highlands Les told me not to worry about anything he would get it sorted out.

That night as I lay in my bed, I couldn't decide who needed who the most, and I was also very scared that I wouldn't fit in a normal house, normal life, for I was far from that. In fact moving away from mad friends, protected places, was not something I had ever really thought about but anyway I soon fell back into my normal day to day life. Mrs Game remarked that Mr Barnes had put in an application for fostering, but nothing else was said life was very hard around here without my soul mate to help me cope, I missed him very much and began to spend an unhealthy time alone, within two weeks I had started another fire at the furthest part of the woods. This time as I stood watching it grew so fast I could feel the power the flames had on me the fire brigade took longer this time to come, and a huge amount of my woods was gone forever. Soon I would have nowhere to hide, for her voice was already sending me quite insane. Away from everyone I would be able to shout back which didn't really do me any good, but it released some anger which was always good but with people around I could only listen to her and her voice grew stronger everyday.

My sixteenth birthday came and went, I was in fact quite depressed by then I had a cake and candles and cards and Les and Pat came in the evening with presents galore but even for them I

could not make myself cheer up. Les went to talk to Janice about me, when at last he returned, he said that the doctor was going to see me tomorrow and he might even give some more pills, to lift the depression that I was in. I knew I was in something I just didn't seem to have any fight in me, I felt like an empty shell.

The following day Dr Woodcock did indeed give me some more pills but more of the same as I was already on. He asked me if I was eating and because I didn't answer him Mrs Game did. She told him that I had not eaten anything properly for nearly a week, so then the doctor went on and on about, how important it was to eat regular meals. I got so fed up I stood up opened the door and took myself back to my room, "fucking stupid bastards the lot of them" I screamed to myself, I wish they would all die.

My lower stomach hurt it was silly cutting myself there, but I did have a very good reason for doing it. I was only trying to cut on top of scars I had already got, well my lower and the top of my legs had still got the scars of my first period, so a few days ago instead of my poor arms I started there. It was not a good place for it hurt every time I moved, not that I really cared, for the more I hurt the more mother stayed away.

I had been to Les and Pat's home for two-week end visits in the last six months. And on a few days out my feelings for them were still very

strong the fostering had gone no where for in two months Les was to retire, and the care authorities declared him too old to foster that hurt him very much. Les tried to find out what was to become off me in the next six months. He was told by someone in the department (who did not wish to be named) that once I reached the age of seventeen, I could do as I wished, for they had no further hold on me, this was just the break Les wanted. So as no laws were being broken Les wanted some papers to be prepared for their signatures and mine to make it legal, so I would be able to live with them. I was starting to worry my self-stupid. Mother had made it very clear that no one was having me. I had spent my entire life being told what to do, how to do it, when to eat, when to sleep, and so on and so on. But in a few months time I would belong to a different world, and that really scared me.

One month later on August the fourth. I was summoned to the office. Woodcock and Mrs Game was in there. They said I had just over a month to run on the care order and if indeed I did still want to live with the Barnes then there would be NO objection. However because of the long period of time I had been institutionalised, they decide for one month I should get the hang of living in the community with a properly registered foster family. I was to leave on Friday. Do you agree to everything I have said asked the doctor? I nodded and asked where the foster family lived. He looked down on his papers and said

"Thundersly" hmm he said "not far from the Barneses" I asked him how far and he thought for a moment and said "about twenty miles or so". As I stood to go the doctor wished me all the luck in the world, and hoped I would find the happiness I deserved, he even shook my hand. As I closed his office door I knew that a new chapter of my life was soon to begin.

Friday came too soon, I would miss all the kids and staff especially Mrs Game, but to be honest it was my woods I would truly yearn for, my time spent in them was my happiest. A lady arrived in a big seven seater her name was Alice. She was very fat. No wonder she had a big car. She came in and had a cup of tea or something. And Mrs Game was giving her papers to sign I in the mean time had gone down the side track and began running for my life for I had to say goodbye to Josh so I had to reach the den. As I sat at the entrance my heart was pounding, I had not ran like that for a long time, I crawled inside and said my goodbyes to a friend I would never forget, after a while I crawled out, stood up and took one last look at my beloved place. With my mood very low I started the walk back to Highlands.

Do you know out of all my different lives this is the one I loved the best? I did not relish the idea of joining the adult race, but at nearly seventeen I had no choice, for it was adults who had inflicted all the pain on me over all these years. As I got back they had only just come out to

find me, we loaded my things in the back and then came the hard bit. I walked over to Mrs Game and told her I would like to say something she nodded so I cleared my throat and began "in my years here I have always found you to be a very fair and decent lady, you care very much about all the kids, a lot more than just doing your job, this family runs well because you are the centre piece, that all the other pieces needed, I have a great deal of respect for you Mrs Game, and I will miss you, thank you for being here for me". She opened her arms and I flung myself into them wishing I could stay forever. As the truck (as I call it) reversed to the corner, I saw Mrs Game wiping her eyes, and we drove off to another life, Alice seemed alright, but something told me that I was not going to like living in a normal family.

The journey took about forty minutes and we pulled down this long road and straight into one of the driveways, I got out of the truck and stared at the height of the house. Alice watched me and said, "yes there is three floors and a lot of stairs", between us we carried the bags to the front door and walked in, leave your bags at the foot of the stairs for now, lets sit and have a nice cup of tea together, and a chat, "sorry" I said "I don't like tea I only drink coffee" she replied" oh do you now, well you wont be getting a lot of that around here, tea is much cheaper, do you think, all the money I get for looking after you, covers coffee and alike, well you will soon see", I looked at her and simply replied " I will have water then".

This was going to be a long four weeks, after she had drunk her tea, she told me to follow her upstairs, she just walked straight passed my bags leaving me to carry them all. Of course my bedroom was on the top floor. We walked into this bedroom. A girl's bedroom, posters on the walls, there was two beds and furniture. I asked which was mine. Oh none of them. That one's Lucy's my eldest daughter. She is fifteen. And that is May's. We adopted her nearly two years ago. Just wait here and I will get you a bed. She came back in with a small put you up bed. The mattress was as thin as toilet paper. And by the time she unfolded it there was no passageway to the other beds. When I said about this. She said, "it was OK the girls will just jump over the bottom of it". Well I will tell you I was not at all impressed. I will get some bedding out for you and off she went. And again she entered the room she threw the bedding onto the bed, and said "I suppose you can make a bed" my face started to red with anger, and I knew I couldn't make trouble in these four weeks, but this was not right. I asked her very politely, why she kept on taking more foster children in when she obviously didn't have the room. This time it was Alice's turn to go red. But maybe she didn't want an argument or maybe she had no answer, because she just turned and went thumping downstairs. I made the bed and as I lay on it the springs kept on moving as I did, I had a lot more comfort in my den than I had here. I started to get my clothes out and realised there was no where to put them. So without delay I skipped down the

stairs and asked Alice where I was to keep my clothes, "in your bag of course" she said, I replied "what all the time" she said "yes your only going to be here for four weeks you can manage that can't you". I left the kitchen I thought "four weeks, too bloody long", Alice came charging through saying "we will have none of that language in this house, we are all God's people here, and while you are here I expect you to obey our rules".

Laying on my camp bed I wished I were back at highlands, I bet it was bloody Woodcock who had chose this set of foster parents for me. I decided after diner I would go to a phone box and ring Les and pat.

About three thirty the noise was out of this world kids running up and down, crying, shouting, how many there was I had no clue, but a bloody lot. Then a big girl walked into my room and then turned around and walked straight out. "Mum" she was shouting down the stairs. At last <u>darling mum</u> yelled back "what?" Lucy yelled "why have you got another one in our room, you said we could have it to ourselves for a while" "yes love, but we needed the money, and it is only for four weeks", (well that made me very welcome). Lucy came in, walked over to the bottom of my bed and started unpacking her school bag. I laid on my bed as I didn't give a shit and started humming, out of the corner of my eyes I could see her doing her home work but well you know me anything for a quiet life, my humming started to get louder when Lucy,

suddenly shouted at me to pack it in. I said, "Sorry are you talking to me, or a bit of shit" she didn't answer so I again started humming, I was very good at winding people up. About thirty seconds later she slammed her books on the bed and climbed over mine and stood right next to me. I said "have you got a problem" she said "yes if you don't stop humming I will bash your head in", that's all I needed, at five foot six inch and about eleven stone, I was more than a match for her, I sat up removed my jumper and stood up. The look in that kid's eye said it all, but I was all fired up now for a fight. Look Lucy said "I'm sorry, I just had a really bad day", "that's OK" I said but you can't talk to a mad girl like me and get away with it. You wanted one now let's get on with it. With that Lucy turned and ran into the hall and bombed it down all those stairs. I fell back on my bed laughing; one down God knows how many more to go.

The little one May. The one they adopted, was a sweet little mite, she was nine, in fact she reminded me of my Lindsay, all except the hair, a number of young boys put their heads in my door to get a look at the mad kid I suppose, I remained upstairs until the bell went. May told me it means we had to go down for dinner? In the front room, come dinning room there were two tables pushed together. A man came from the TV room and said "hello I'm George, head of the house hold, its nice to have you at our table", we all sat, and Alice started to bring the food in, egg on toast I looked

at it but didn't understand why we were not having a proper meal, all eight kids with me got egg on toast, but George and Alice had a stew, with dumplings and potatoes. All the kids had their heads bowed and George began prayers, "fuck this for a game of soldiers", I thought. Well you know me, never knew when to keep my mouth shut. I asked Alice politely why did all the children have egg on toast, when they both had a descent meal. George said "I will answer that luv, you see Lindsay all the children have school dinners, so they don't require another meal, where myself and Alice work all day, and just have a sandwich, does that answer your question". Well yes, but I am not at school, so I will not get a diner from there. So I suppose I will get my diner as well in the evening. "NOT LIKELY" Alice answered; "money is hard enough to go round you will eat what the rest of the children in this family eat. Like it or lump it."

It was very obvious that these people didn't care about the children; I think they were in for the money. After so called diner I told them I was going out for a walk. Alice said "don't take all night over it" as I closed the front door I felt nothing, but loathing for these people I had to find a phone box and phone Les. I found one near some shops, and I phoned his number. Les answered and knew there was something wrong. He told me to give him the phone number of the phone box, which I did and he told me he would ring straight back. I started to tell him about what had been happening. Firstly he was appalled at the fact I

was on a camp bed and the dinner well that made him really angry, also the fact I could not drink coffee. He told me not to worry, that he would get it sorted out for me. There was no way he was letting me stay there, but I had to promise that I would not do anything bad. He told me to ring him at one o'clock the next day; I told him I could not take four weeks of this. And he said, "He would get it sorted".

As I walked back, I felt a lot better as Les had never let me down before. True to his word about eleven o'clock the next morning a lady came, I could hear Alice's voice getting louder, then two sets of footsteps on the stairs, I remained laying on the camp bed. This posh lady took two steps into the room, for anymore she would be standing on me. She tooted then asked Alice to go back down stairs, as she wanted a word with me in private. As she went we heard her say "she is nothing but a trouble maker". The lady, Julie asked me a lot of things and I told her the truth about the drinks, dinner, my bed, and nowhere to put my clothes and the way Alice spoke to me. I told her I phoned my new foster dad last night, because I felt this was all wrong, I also told her that Alice would make my mental illness worse Julie looked around the bed room and agreed I could not be expected to live in these conditions. She told me to pack. With that I laughed, for everything was in my bags from yesterday. She asked me to remain upstairs until she called me. With that Julie went down stairs, I could hear

Alice's voice, not Julie's and she was not too happy. I remained upstairs for about an hour. Then Julie came up and helped me carry my bags down. The front door was ajar and as Julie and I walked through it, who was waiting on the other side for me? "Dad I shouted as I ran into his open arms", its all right kid you're coming home. Dad thanked the lady, as so did I. We both drove off to our new life together; we were like little kids on how we had done it. I tell you this, my dad is a very clever man, as we both calmed down Les turned to me and said "do you know the best part of all this" you called me dad, and that makes me feel so proud. "Is it alright then?" I asked. "All right, it is more than all right, it's bloody fantastic."

I had never had a dad or a daddy. Or a mum and mummy. And they were a different breed of people for all these were kind, loving and cherished their children, where as mothers and fathers used them, for their own mad way of life, to rape them and give them so much pain that they wanted to die, for these people were sick.

Finally we got home and unloaded my bags, I asked "where Pat was" dad said "she's at work", we walked in and at that very moment I knew I was home. Dad and I carried my bags upstairs. And went back down to put the kettle on, dad looked at me sitting at the table with a grin on his face "I suppose you want coffee" I burst out laughing so did dad he told me it was going to be great having me around. For Pat still worked and

he got a bit lonely sometimes. As we drank, I asked him did Pat know I am home for good, "no" he said, "that's your surprise for her". I sat thinking and asked if he picked her up from work "yes" he said she can't drive, so my plan came out. Dad lent me some money and we went to the flower shop. I picked out this beautiful bunch of flowers, and I asked them to wrap them for me they gave me a card to write on. But we took it home so as to have more time to think what to write.

Dad said put "to mum I'm home for good", my face went as white as a cloud "what's up kid?" dad asked, I can't call her that, you don't understand, he got out of his chair and knelt beside me and asked "what didn't I understand" in very short and quick way told him that mother had beaten me and my stepfather had abused me, and I really didn't want to go into it yet. He cradled my head to his chest and said "it's all right we have the rest of our lives to talk about it" and I know Pat will understand. So, on the card I put dear Pat, hope you still love me for you have got me for the rest of your life.

The journey to the supermarket was very exciting, dad was going as he always did and I was to hide behind the car, and jump out on her. It seemed never ending, but as I sat I saw them coming, just as she was about to open the door, I jumped out, and it scared her. But soon she was all over me, saying what was I doing here. I gave her my flowers and told her to read the card. She

read my words out loud and dropped the flowers and gave me a cuddle that I would never forget. She picked her flowers up and there in the supermarket car park we hugged and kissed like never before, for my new life had begun. Finally I had a family who LOVED ME.

Chapter Eleven

These two wonderful people took a young disturbed tearaway into their home, and their hearts gave me love, more than any real parent could have given. I thanked God that in this world that there are still people like mine around. For all they asked of me back, was to love them, and to learn, to love myself.

Within a week I told dad I wanted to find a job, he asked me, didn't I want time to settle down first, but I could not tell him that I was feeling a bit smothered, I just wasn't used to all this love and kindness. We agreed to start looking. Dad took me around newsagent's windows and he bought the local papers, I didn't know what sort of job I even wanted. But I did know I wanted to be outside. Friday evening we picked Pat up from work, after diner I sat looking through the job adds, "there it was". Farm hand wanted pigs unit, must be fit and willing to work long hours, and some weekends, phone 0916-77654, evenings. I showed dad, he could feel the excitement in me, "are you sure kid?" he said, "yes" I replied "there's the phone ring them". So I did. I spoke to the boss Mr Lang. He told me that it was hard physical work, but if I thought I could do it, to go at nine thirty for an interview, as I put the phone down I punched the air with my fist, and said "yes".

Mr Lang. was a middle aged fat man, bald, and very well spoken, as we spoke he looked me

up and down, he showed me around the farm, (oh the smell) four to five thousand pigs he owned, it was a breeding farm, pigs coming and going all the time. He asked if I could drive, I said "no but in two weeks I will be old enough to get my licence, and my dad is going to teach me straight away", I could tell by his face that he needed someone who could drive, but I <u>wanted</u> this job, and I was not going to lose it, I told him to put me on a months trial, if it didn't work out. He would have not lost anything. He said "he liked my spirit, and he could see I would be able to handle the hard work, so <u>yes</u> he would give me a trial". We walked into his office and he told me the wages and hours, plus you would work every other weekend. I offered my hand to him as we parted and told him that he would not regret this, as I turned to walk to the car he said "I forgot to tell you there are four men working here, so expect a few jokes". "Don't worry Mr Lang I can handle myself", I said and I heard him say, "I bet you can". I jumped into dad's car and told him to drive, when we were far enough away, I shouted yippee. Dad was really pleased Pats worried it would be too hard for me, I, well I saw it as way of being free. I explained everything that was said I thought dad might be angry about the driving bit, but instead he started making plans for him to give me lessons.

They were both pleased about the wages of twenty-seven pounds and fifty pence take home it was good for a first job. We all sat at the table making lists of what I needed and transport to the

farm; it was a little over a mile from home. I could bike it in ten minutes, and on a rainy day dad would take me. I was at last going to join the human race, that afternoon dad and me went to town dad got me a pair of green overalls, green Wellingtons, lunch box, a flask and a back pack to carry them in.

Monday seven thirty am. Dad brought me down in his car to work, holding my back pack I walked into the farm office Mr Lang said "good morning" and introduced me to the farm manager Phil, and to the three farm hands Ben, Alan, Wayne they jeered at me. I will admit I was shitting bricks but only on the inside, on the outside I was cool, calm and collective. For the first day I was at work with Phil he would go through the feeding, mucking out and breeding (BREEDING YOU MUST BE JOKING) in fact that would become my responsibility, for each worker had a section that they were responsible for. I couldn't get over the sheer size and weight of some of the animals. And the noise in the first hour was enough to burst your eardrums. For I had ninety percent of the adult pigs, and everyone of them wanted feeding first Phil was very nice he explained it all as we did it, but he did give me a very important piece of advice that I was never to forget. The female pigs (sows) could live together quite happily but, and he meant BUT you must never put two boars (males) together for they would fight to the death. Boars have big tusks and they're bigger and stronger than any female, **always be on your**

guard, never turn your back on them. I told him that I would always remember what he had said. My day in the life as a pig farmer was cankering. After bathing and my dinner I fell asleep on the settee. But today I had fulfilled a dream for I worked alongside normal people No Homes, No Psychiatric Homes, No Mental Hospitals, No Adolescence Homes, No Foster Homes, today I was normal and to be working outside was my greatest pleasure of all. I even had to admit the pigs were not bad either, once you got to know them.

During my first week the lads did indeed play some tricks on me, the first was killing a rat, cutting its guts open then tying it up by its legs to the rafters of the feed block. So when I come in it came down straight in my face, I tell you it scared the shit out of me. Next one I had been shown how to drive a mucking out tractor, and the seat was always wet so you had to put a meal sack on it so as your arse did not get wet. Well that morning there was already a sack on it, so off I went to muck my sows out Unbeknown to me that the sack was filled with dead rats. (Although I had not yet got my driving licence, because we were on private land I could drive). I took many tricks in the first few weeks there but I didn't respond to any of them and they soon stopped.

Today I got my first pay packet although it was the end of my second week; I had to work a week in hand. Mr Lang gave it to me and said, "so

far he was very pleased with my work". All the way home I kept looking at it I had never had that much money before in my life, and I had earned it. That evening I asked dad and Pat how much they would like for my keep each week. Dad said "nothing it is yours to keep". Pat said "that was up to me". I asked if seven pounds and fifty pence was enough she said "more than enough" I also told them that each time I got a raise or bonus that I would give them half of what I got extra. They said I was very thoughtful and they were proud of me for sticking to my job, especially how tired I was all the time. In two days time it was my birthday, dad had all the forms all done and ready to post for my provisional driving licence, for driving a tractor at work, had really made me want to drive dad's car.

My birthday came and went, I was really too tired to enjoy it, we went out to a restaurant for dinner, for like I say it was nothing special.

My trial passed and I was given a contract to say I became a fully-fledged farm hand. Days rolled into weeks, weeks into months, and like a bad penny always turns up, so mothers voice returned, stronger, more determined than ever before. Mother made my days a nightmare, and my bad dreams returned I had moved on from hurting myself for I was no longer a child, so how does an adult cope with MOTHER. I decided that mother was not going to make me lose every thing that I had earned and worked for, so for the first

time in my life, I told dad everything about my life. He cried in places, he hugged me asking why I had not told him any of this before, I explained about Arthur, William, and my Lindsay and last of all MOTHER.

He cuddled me and kissed me for he understood why I had never told a soul. To protect my brother was my only goal. He asked me why I had told him now. He asked was I in trouble I said "yes". I told him I was in danger of losing him and Pat. And also my job he said "Lindsay you listen to me nothing do you hear me, nothing is ever going to split our family up". I asked him if we could keep all this to our selves, I didn't want Pat to know for I had broken my wall of silence to him because I knew he would honour my wishes. He agreed as I knew he would I told him about mothers voice hounding me and he came up with an idea. He told me to wear my headphones that way mother's voice could not get in, what I didn't know was If I could wear them for work.

I tried dad's headphones and nearly got run over by a bloody tractor for I had tried having them on full volume, so that idea couldn't be used at work anyway. Dad came up with more things singing to myself, that didn't work kept forgetting the words because mother was shouting above me all the time I am afraid nothing we did stopped her. I hadn't told dad about the self-harm, it had worked before, quite frankly I was desperate to try anything. With one of dad's disposable razors, I

cut my arms to pieces I didn't hurt, not while I was doing it anyway. I think my body was so used to pain that I could just block it out. For nearly a month I carried on scaring my body, it helped but not as much as when I was a child, the reason was soon to become clear. That amount of pain was a child's answer, but now an adult child's pain was not enough. **I would have to think bigger.**

While I sat in the park, swallowing the pills with a beer I knew that I would lose everything, but there was no answer. I convinced myself that it was better to have loved and lost than never to have loved at all. When my debt had been done. I went home to die. I lay in my bed and wrote dad and Pat a letter. Thanking them for showing me what it was like to be part of a real family. As I wrote tears fell on the page, why was this world such a cruel place for here I am, a new family great job, I should be as happy as Larry but NO mother has taken all that away from me. I had become weak I was like putty in her hands.

Dad was shaking me "what have you taken Lindsay tell me" dad was rubbing my head and arms as he was saying "Lindsay we need to know what you have taken". The next thing I knew I had a mask over my face I was in a white room, "Lindsay's room" no I cant be in Lindsay's room I thought mother was yelling SILLY BITCH CAN`T EVEN KILL HERSELF over and over she was repeating her words I looked around, I was in hospital, "STOP IT" I screamed "STOP IT", but

she just carried on repeating herself finally I passed out. At last I was at peace.

I awoke in a single room for a moment I thought I was back at Grasslands mental hospital, for it was very similar I got out of bed, I had a white gown on with ties at the back I walked to the open door, and stared in pure disbelief up and down the corridor were patients. Some standing still, some walking, it took just one look to tell me I was mad again. I slid down the wall and sat on my arse in pure disbelief. Two nurses came one each side of me, picked me up frog marched me back into my room. They dressed me in a top and trousers, (like prison uniform) and then marched me to a room full of high-backed chairs. There I was left to get on with it. I remained on Firland Ward for thirty-three days, dad and Pat visited but most of the time my mind was else where. On the thirty fourth-day dad picked me up and together with a bag full of pills I went home.

Being home and flushing my pills I soon began to be myself again. Dad had told Mr Lang that I had to have an operation so my job was still there for me. Within four days of being home I started back with my pigs again. Mother kept away for a nice long time, and I soon returned to normal. I often spoke of my love for a dog of my own, I mean I loved animals my job proved that, but the farm was not a safe place to have pets running around. Pat was not any animal lover, but it would be nice for dad to have company for the day.

Anyway as I said I had spoken a few times but with no response so I gave up.

This weekend was my weekend off on Saturday morning dad asked if I would like to go into town, (well I am a typical woman, and I love shopping). So off I drove with dad to town I was becoming quite a good driver I suppose, because dad was an excellent teacher. We parked and dad started walking, he said he just needed to get a few things first can you bare with me. A few streets later we walked into the pet shop dad stood in all his glory looking at the cages as I looked I could see there was a litter of puppies in the big cage I looked at dad and he smiled and said "pick one kid". Well I can't tell you the feelings I had; it was like nothing on earth, I looked at all these tongues and noses and I was as happy as I had ever been in my life. Dad and I were looking at them when I heard a whimper from a cage at the top, I could see a black nose, and I just about managed to reach up and touch it. The puppy was whimpering and when I took my hand away, it started to wail really loud so I got the steps that was in the corner of the shop, and stood on them to reveal a black and white head, with small ears and a really long tongue, she licked my fingers and pressed her warm body up to the side of the cage. As I got down I told dad that's the pup I wanted. He said, "You can't even see it properly". But one look at my face was enough to answer his question. The shop owner said "that he had sold her in a litter about three months ago, and that the

woman had brought her back to the shop saying her and her husband had split up and that she could not look after the dog on her own". He said he didn't even know how she was; I told him none of it mattered that we would give her a good home. He told us to step back and as he opened the cage she jumped straight into my arms. I don't know who was more shocked the shopkeeper or me. She was licking my face and biting my nose, she was just so excited, her long skinny tail was going around and around in circles. I knew that we were made for each other. Dad and the shopkeeper watched, as me and my pup loved each other. Dad bought her a collar and lead, toys, bowls, treats and a basket, it came to a great deal of money, but he knew she would be worth every penny. I carried her to the car; dad carried all her things. He told me the shopkeeper was so over come that he did not charge dad for the pup. He told him it was like watching a match made in heaven. Dad said I had to do everything for her and to make sure I cleaned up after her, I promised that I would. I asked him did Pat know he said yes but it had taken quite a while to persuade her. Dad drove, I sat on the back seat with my puppy on my lap, and she soon went fast to sleep. What shall I call her I asked dad, "I don't know" he said, "it's up to you". At home she loved the garden, God could she run, dad thinks she has some whippet in her, or terrier, or maybe collie. She was a right Heinz fifty-seven. We placed her basket in the corner of the kitchen, we put a water bowl down for her, we had not got any dog food

yet, we would get it when we picked Pat up at lunch time. My puppy's lead and collar is red she didn't like the collar, she kept on trying to get it off, I ran up and down the garden with her wherever I went she followed. At that time we used to watch the TV programme called Mork and Mindy day suggested we call her Mindy so from that day on her name was Mindy. Pat soon fell in love with her she was that sort of dog, she had a basket in the kitchen but night she slept in bed with me. Winter or summer she always slept under the covers, Mindy was a law unto herself, when I took her to the park I would walk straight across the field not Mindy she always went around the edges.

One day Pat said to me "do you realise that since Mindy's been sleeping with you, that you had no bad dreams". I think having her I had learnt the true feeling of love, for I loved every hair on her body. At weekends I took her to the farm with me to work but it didn't workout because she kept on barking at the pigs. My life carried on and with my new best friend I had a very good reason not to take anymore pills, for now I didn't have my self to think about I had my four legged friend.

For about the next three years or so my life on the whole was good. I passed my driving test and bought my very own, old banger it was a white mini traveller. Mindy and me went everywhere in it, I kept the back seats folded down with a blanket over them so as on long journeys Mindy could lay down and sleep. It was nice not

getting up, so early for work having my car also meant that at lunch times, I could come home to dad, who would have something hot waiting for me, also in those three years Mr Lang made me under manager to Phil, I got a nice wage increase not that the lads were happy, but I was. I put one hundred and one percent into my job, more than I can say for most. Dad got me some books from the library and he would help me read and understand them. I formed a friendship that had become an important part of my learning progress. A boar who was there when I started working at the farm had become a very good friend to me, "yes laugh if you want". But Prince as I named him, was different from the others, he was black and white, large, very hairy but with a very laid back attitude to life. I remember my manager Phil calling him "a bit of a drip". But they were wrong, I know my friendship to him, was food, because that's all any of the farm animals thought about. But for me it was a lot more. Boars could kill; they had tusks that could rip your legs open, and a real mean temper, but not <u>Prince</u>. He was different, as our friendship grew; I could sit on the straw in his pen scratching his back. He would lick food from my hands. I found later on, that I could sit on his back, and he would walk around his enclosure quite happily, we really had formed a bond. I trusted him and he me. I told Prince things, that I could never tell a person, he became someone to trust, not because he couldn't talk but the peace and calm that came from him. Every evening before going home I never failed to say goodnight

(and leave him a bit of supper). The lads found out and for a long time, I was the topic of the jokes, but that never bothered me, I had broad shoulders our friendship was more important than that.

Mindy had grown into a beautiful dog "but God did she have a mind of her own" in our house dad made a sign "Mindy rules OK". Oh but how we all loved her, she was so stubborn, if she didn't want to do or go somewhere, there was no making her, short of carrying her of course, but that's what made her so different. More so to dad, but he spent the most time with her. One day out walking I lost her, "the panic" I felt was the same as when I was a child I ran up and down the same piece of beach, a hundred times, calling her name. I was and looked like a "mad woman", but fear had really grabbed me. After I don't know how long I ran all the way home, crying as I was going. Dad and me got into his car, and drove back to where I last saw her. We both searched in different directions, but she was nowhere to be seen. Dad said, "We should go home", just in case she has but I felt like I was giving up. In the end of hours of searching we drove home, as dad pulled into our drive, we saw Mindy sitting on the front doorstep. Our hearts filled with joy, but dad, as well as, me got out and were telling her what a naughty girl she was, but at the same time cuddling her, we both aged that day. I think it really makes you appreciate what you have got, when you think you have lost it for I am sure, for if at possible, I loved Mindy more from that day on.

I decided I wanted a motorbike, like all good parents Pat tried to talk me out of it but not dad, he told Pat to let me make my own mind up, I was no longer a child, so yes of course, dad and me went around all the bike shops. I wanted a brand new one, so that's what I got (on hp of course). A Suzuki 50cc trials bike, red, oh she was a beauty, I got a leather bike jacket and a crash helmet, gloves and other bits and pieces. Because I now earned at least two hundred and fifty pounds a month, getting hp was no problem, dad signed as well and my bike was delivered within a week. I suppose it took about a week or so until I felt comfortable to ride to work on it, but I went all over the place on her in fact I sold my old mini a short time later.

One day just out of the blue, without thinking about it I called Pat, Ma, I realised what I had said when Pat said "that's nice I like that". So did I, thought so from that day on, Pat was my Ma, I never forgot from one day to another, how lucky I was to have them, they support me and love me without any condition.

During this period of time my voices, came and went, never any pattern to her anger, but I had learnt a way to control her, not totally, but quite a lot. Mindy gave me the answer, the way she always walked the sameway, stopped at the same places, she always did things the same; I started very slowly at first to do mothers jobs her

way. (I will try to explain) before work, I made my bed and examined it the same way as I did as a child for mother, then it seemed that mother was not so mad at me. It started with my bed and within a year I was doing things so different, it was controlling my days, but it was worth it, like I said "I've not been ill for a long time". Dad saw what was going on and kept on telling me it was not the right thing, "but he was wrong", for I was better, (or was I?). If only when this started I had told dad, he would have stopped me before I got this far, for now I could never stop. I was being controlled through mother, I had given her tools to make my life hell even more, but I had to carry on, for if I had ever stopped she would make me pay. I started to count how many times I had washed my hands, I counted steps, seconds, spoonfuls, Mindy's steps the list was endless, and as you might guess, I soon ended up back on Firland Ward, at the mental hospital this time I had a total breakdown. Three and a half years after my last admission, I was back. I had not taken pills or anything. I just couldn't function. My brain was knackered, with all the counting. I had remained in hospital for three months but in my time here I had realised what I had done to myself. Mother didn't do it, I did. I convinced myself by doing all these things that mother was happier, and that my voices were quieter of course I was very wrong, but once I started I couldn't stop. Mrs Jones, No Dr Jones my quack on the ward, understood what I had done to myself, and why. She had told me what Dr Woodcock had said all those years

before, that I have a split personality, two people in one, and that I would not probably be any different. And that I would have to live with mother's voice, but not to let her control me. That her voice alone could not hurt me, that I had to learn to stop listening to her. I explained that I had, mother within me for ten years. And that I had never learned how to stop listening to her, Dr Jones told me that with medication, I could live a reasonable quality of life, I felt because she seemed to know what I was suffering that I would give her pills a go.

I remained off work so long I had to hand in my notice. For the doctors had told me. I would not be fit enough to return for at least six months. Although I had been signed off I knew Mr Lang, would need to fill my place so now because off my own stupidity, I had lost my job of four years with beloved Prince. I felt very hollow, for I really believe, by living like I was it was going to rid me of mother, how stupid could I be. I was twenty one years old, no job, a shadow of my former self I had lost so much weight for I never had time to eat, dad felt bad for he knew what I was doing, but he didn't think it was out of control. He, like me, would have tried anything to make me normal.

It was taking the pills and being with dad and Mindy I started to eat and get my strength back. Dad was the best medicine anyone could wish for, he loved me so much I knew if need be, he would die for me. I returned to see Dr Jones

three months after my release and she was amazed on how different I looked, she told me I would have to take the pills for the rest of my life, but as I told her, it would be a small price to pay for being happy. When she asked had the voices gone completely I replied "yes" which was a big mistake. I thought if I told the truth, she would have put me back on the ward, and that's the last thing I wanted. Truthfully mother was still with me, but controllable, I parted saying "thank you very much I hope I don't see you again" lying with ease I had done it enough.

About a few weeks later I was riding my bike on country roads, and going round a sharp bend, an on coming car knocked me off my bike. I laid in the road the pain in my legs were really bad. Someone was talking to me but I still had my full-face helmet on. The words were muffled, I was trying to undo my strap when a face appeared in my visor, a man lifted my visor up and told me not to move, and to leave my helmet on until the ambulance arrived. "My bike" I said "sorry lad it's all busted up" "I'm not a lad I'm a woman" I said quite angrily, "sorry" he said. It's all the leather gear. Are you in great pain he asked? I replied "it was my leg". And he said "it was bent" the ambulance arrived, blue lights, and all they put was a big collar on me and removed my helmet, I was so relieved to get it off, they put padding and straps on my leg, and gave me oxygen to breath. The man was very worried, I asked him if he could phone my dad and let him know what had

happened, he said, "he would" I gave him the number as I was being lifted into the ambulance.

I had already been to x-ray when dad and ma had arrived at the hospital; they were both in a state. Ma kept on saying "I did not want her to have that bloody bike in the first place; I knew something like this would happen". Dad looked at me and said "are you alright kid" "yes I have just broke my leg" "just broke your leg" ma was really weird. This young doctor came with my x-ray in his hand, he explained my leg was fractured, but that it had already been broken before, and had not been noticed, he asked me if many years earlier, had I broken it and had it in plaster. I said "no". Dad asked to speak to him in private and the both left, of course I know what he meant. He meant that mother had beaten me so badly, of course my leg could have been broken, dad knew that as well as I did, we sat waiting for dad to return, I was praying dad was not saying anything he shouldn't, dad soon returned. I would have to be put out and then they could re-break the old one and reset them both together. I asked why they had to re-break the old one, but dad explained that the two brakes were on the same bone. The doctor told him he didn't know how leg had never given me any trouble, he said "it was one for the books", dad told me I had to stay in for a few days and be in plaster for six weeks. "My bike" I said "dad what about my bike" "don't worry kid I will get it sorted".

Of course he did, my bike was taken to the insurance people, about two months later I got a cheque for six hundred and fifty pounds a fortune, well for me, by then my cast had come off, I could never use them bloody crutches, in fact I could walk quite well, Mindy never complained.

I was as well as I could ever be, and started to get bored, it was time to find another job, "**BUT WHAT**", for weeks I looked in the papers, asked around, all that was about was shop work, I couldn't do that, I looked in all the shop windows, nothing. Ma said, "Shop work's not that bad", I have done it for twenty years, anyway she said "it will do you for now". The next day I went to our local co-op and applied for the job, filling the forms out there and then. I was told to come for an interview on Friday at ten fifteen am. As I walked home all I could think about were the farm and my Prince, I was not looking forward to Friday, for working indoors was no life for me.

Yes I know, I got the bloody job and the bloody uniform, I was not looking forward to Monday for my life is outside not in.

Chapter Twelve

The co-op opened a New World for me that I never knew that was there. In my whole life, I had had worlds that I would study, and watch, 'til I knew all the people in them and their ways, but the co-op and its world, was so vast, I felt lost in the sea of people. In all the homes, hospital units, etc, the people were few. And hardly ever changed, even the farm, but now, here I was overcome with all the faces. I didn't feel safe and in control, but I knew I had to learn to be a person, like all the rest. I felt lonely and sometimes frightened by all the faces and my eyes, that I didn't know "were they evil? Or kind" too many for me, to try and judge. Those few days were the hardest in my life. Dad understood, he said "I had been institutionalised so much, but that it would do me good, to see the world. For what it really was, of course like always he was right. My work was boring, I never had a very good brain, but for all this work you didn't need one. I found a friend amongst the staff, she was a loner like me, her name was, Andrea Woods, and we were both on the same shifts together. It started very slowly, we would have our lunch together, then we started to walk part of the way home together, I enjoyed her company, she had few friends because she believed she was fat, ugly, and uninteresting, and so on. I felt I could relate to her, (I didn't find her any of those things, in fact quite the reverse). Dad was so pleased, he encourages me to go out and see how I would get on, outside the co-op walls.

This Friday we made plans to visit our local pub together, just for an hour or so. Andrea was so used to staying in the safety of her parent's four walls that this outing was indeed, as a bigger thing for her as it was for me.

Next day the manager asked to see me in his upstairs office, although I had done nothing wrong that I knew of, but it was liked being summoned by one of the quacks at the unit. I stood in front of Mr Wise and trembled he explained that he wanted someone to join the team of people working on the delicatessen, and that he would like it to be me, I would have less contact with the public, and more preparation work to do, he explained that hams, cheese, bacon and meats etc. all came to the store in a bulk, then in the rooms behind the deli they were cut and prepared, "would you like to have a go" oh yes he said "it's twenty one pence per hour more" what about it? "Yes" I said "I`LL give it a go." The less I contact with the public would suit me down to the ground plus more money. I had a darker top than the shop floor people and a name badge. And within two days, I was indeed a lot happier, I was away from the sea of people, and I even enjoyed getting all the food ready to be served on the counter.

It's Friday night and I am already, in my jeans and my new jumper to face the pub. Dad told me to enjoy myself and to loosen up, we met at Andréa's house. As we walked to the red lion, I

don't know who was the most scared as we entered the pub. I had been elected to get the first drinks. We stayed about one and half-hours, and the music, and the chatter and drink made it quite a nice evening. Walking home we both decided, we would like to do it every Friday, after I walked Andrea home, I returned home feeling a lot more positive about myself, than I had felt in a long time. Having a friend like Andrea would be very good for me (well for both of us really).

I actually enjoyed work now, being behind the scenes was so much easier for me, I even made another friend, her name was Jane Weaver, she was a quite a bit younger than me, but I did in fact like her very much, she was a shelf filler, so she was able to pop into my room a lot, on and of during the day she was like my "little ray of sunshine". Jane saw good in everyone, she was so sensitive and innocent but I did enjoy her company very much, for in Jane I saw an older Lindsay.

"Look at me" I have a new job, friends and getting out, it was enough to make any body think I was a normal woman, "except dad of course", for only he could see my fight with mother still going on. The pills helped, I'm sure they did because I seemed to be in control, well most of the time. I had unbeknown to anyone, returned to some "<u>only some</u>" of my old ways, that kept "mother calm", Mindy had given me the answer from day one. To only walk "the walk"? To never step out of the

walk. To always to stay in the safe areas. I had six walks that I knew all the steps to. As long as I <u>not Mindy</u>, stayed in the boundaries. Mother remained calm. By getting dressed and undressed exactly the right way and order. Mother remained calm there was in fact quite a few things more, but they are more personal I have indeed in my life time had tried many ways to please mother, and this restricted way of life, seemed to help the most.

Andrea gave me these papers today at work, on going abroad, on three to four day trips, she asked if I would go on one with her, I told her I would look at it my dad was over the moon "go for it kid", was his answer. Ma was more reserved in fact her answer was "what about your pills", well you know me it did it, me and Andrea went off to Brussels for three days and nights, in three weeks time. Dad's got me a yearly passport, and changed one hundred pounds from my savings for me. For the first time in my life I would be on my own. Andrea knew nothing of my other life, for if she did I know that I would lose her. I don't remember dad being so happy for me, he said "it's a new beginning for me, to learn to take control of my own life", if only he had known what I had been doing all these months, to keep mother calm. (The fact that I was on the pills during the time did not enter my head).

On the morning of our adventure at five thirty am. Dad took Andrea and me to the main bus station where he put us on our coach to

Brussels, as he cuddled me good bye, we both had tears, for it was the first time we were apart in years. I was sick on the ferry, and for the rest of our coach journey I felt really rough. Our hotel was out of this world, our double room was massive, and we both felt like queens. There was a bar, but dad had warned me not to get anything from it, because it was really expensive, during our time there, we spent a lot of it shopping. One night we went to a local bar, but we soon left because to me it seemed to me it was like they were all talking about us. We went on a lift up the side of this great mountain, it was then I realised I didn't like heights; Andrea took the mickey out of me something chronic, but not in a nasty way. Do you know we had a really good time and although mother was with us she made no trouble?

Dad was over the moon to see us, the fact that I had phoned each day made no difference, on our way home in the car, and he wanted to know everything. We took Andrea home first, then we went home, and Mindy wet herself in the hall, because she was so pleased to see me. I then had to go through it all again for ma. But not with the same zest as for dad, I learnt a very important lesson that week, for I had done something I would have never thought possible, and why, because I took the chance that mother would not rear her ugly head.

Work carried on the same, a few weeks ago Jane and I (my little friend from the co-op)

went to the pictures, then a burger place afterwards, she was a real fun girl and I enjoyed her company a lot. Andrea and me kept going to the Red Lion and had become regulars; we found out that each year all the pubs had a fun day to raise money for charity. This year it was "it's a knock out" and yes you are right, Andrea and me got roped in for it. There were seven different pub teams, and they had set out different races and games on the school fields, it was all just for fun, Andrea kept on and on she didn't want to do it, I knew why because it was shorts and tee-shirts it didn't matter how many times I and others told her she was not fat, she didn't believe us. Anyway in the end she did indeed join in, and play. "It's a knock out" it was fantastic and we came third, in one game the women had to sit in wheel barrows, carrying a full bucket of water, while being pushed over a bumpy course by the men, you can imagine where most of the water ended up. The whole day was really great fun, and me and Andrea, looked forward to the following years, I can't remember how much we made for charity, but it was a lot.

Dad's health is not very good at the moment, the GP put him on even more drugs, and I know it is because he smokes. But I can't say anything because about a few years ago I had started, dad assures me that once the new pills kick in he would be fine, and that's good enough for me.

I am doing more and more things to keep mother happy, I almost go into autopilot, when I am doing them. Ma is getting fed up with me keep-moving things to keep mother happy. Dad then realised that I had started to get out of control again. And unbeknown to me he phoned Dr Jones, on Firland Ward and asked if she could increase my pills. Whether it was that dad was a nurse or what. But she left dad a prescription on the ward. For him to pick up to increase my pills from 20mg twice a day to 30mg twice a day, on the understanding that if in a few weeks I had not started to improve that he would bring me in to see her.

At home after work dad sat me down and explained what he had done. I was angry; he had gone behind my back. I wasn't ill I was fine, just because I liked things neat and tidy even as I was shouting all this to dad. I knew he was right. I <u>was</u> letting her take over me. I cried in my dad's arms and said, "I didn't know of any other way of controlling her voice". Like many times before dad kept on saying, "that's what the pills are for", but like always I knew that it was a lie. "Pills a few pills", how the hell can they help, **"STOP MOTHER"** dad asked me if I trust him? I said "of course I do" then do it now its not all your counting, making everything straight, walking one way, its none of it, "please kid, I love you" it's the pills that make her voice go away. Please trust me. Now the doctor has increased them, within a few days you will be alright. I looked at my dad's

face and I knew I had to say, "Yes I thought he was right" but to say it, and to believe it, and know it, are very different things.

I think dad willed me so much. That indeed in about a week or so I started to feel better, one by one I started not to do all my jobs, but I only stopped the newest ones, I carried on the important ones, out of fear really, not fear of mother but fear of getting ill. Going back to the hospital for I had so much to lose, for the first time in my twenty-three years "I was enjoying my life".

One day a friend of dads came into the co-op, she asked to see me she told me her grandson had just started work on a farm over Meadow Brook Way and they were looking for someone to run their sheep herd. Well she knew I was looking for farm work again and wondered if I was interested. I told her that it was over a year ago that I had been looking, but I would like to go and see what the job entailed. She gave me a piece of paper and said, "The owners Mr and Mrs Hall were very nice people and that her grandson was very happy there. I thanked her very much and went back to my job cutting cheese. I looked at the paper Mr and Mrs Hall, Meadow Brook Way, Lagford, 0125-3863. I put it back in my pocket and spent the rest of my shift dreaming. I was like a kid again. I ran most of the way home. What would dad think? Dad said much the same as I had. That I wouldn't lose anything by going to have a look. As I dialled the number I felt very

nervous, why I don't know but after talking two other people I finally spoke to Mrs Hall she explained, that the sheep herd and a large bird breeding programme was hers, and the farm was run by her husband. Mrs Hall asked me if I would like to go and meet her and see what the job entailed. I will admit I liked the sound of it very much. I explained about the pig farm, and told her I was now working in side, which did not suit me. We then arranged to meet on Monday afternoon at three o'clock. As I put the phone down I felt an air of excitement run through me a thrill I had not had for a long time.

Ma didn't feel that excitement at all her answer to me was if it's not broke don't fix it. But all of a sudden, I felt that same urge for my outside job. The co-op had done so much for me but I never had any joy in my steps going to work. I loved animals with such an inner heart that even the dirtiest jobs never put me off. Dad saw just what a phone call did to me and encouraged me to go for it. I felt on edge right up until dad drove me down the half-mile lane to Meadow Brooke farm. The farm house was massive it was so big it just made me more scared as I walked up to the big front door, it opened and two spaniels came running out and jumped all over me. Mrs Hall stood watching as I fussed over them, she had a smile on her face which was very welcoming, in fact liked her from that very moment. I was invited in to have tea and go through what the job on offer entailed. Do you know sometimes when you have

only just met someone and yet you know you're going to be friends, well that's just how I felt, drinking coffee and talking, we talked for ages. The job was like nothing I had done before, but that didn't seem to bother her. She explained that she had phoned David Lang at Mill Green Farm, and that he had given me an excellent reference, he had also told her not to let me go, that she wouldn't get a better dedicated worker than me. I knew that I blushed; feel my face burning; I also felt proud of myself. We walked the two fields that her four hundred and fifty sheep herd were grazing in. I felt really stupid the fact that I knew nothing about sheep, but it didn't seem to matter, she just kept on saying "you'll soon learn", I knew the job was mine if I wanted it. When Mrs Hall showed me her birds I stood opened mouthed I couldn't believe my eyes, huge man made ponds three of them, all running into each other water falls and hundreds and hundreds of ducks, geese and swans all different colours and sizes. It was an unbelievable sight, Mrs hall explained that she bred them and shipped the young back to their countries of origin. To stop them becoming endangered, also that she did not make it common knowledge that the birds was here, because people might try and steal some of the rarest one simply for their value. I think she could read my mind, for she suddenly said "I have been breeding birds for eighteen years and there are a lot of things I still don't know but believe me its really fun learning". As we walked across to dad's car she took my arm and asked "well the jobs

yours if you want it, I can see you're the sort of person I need for I can see you have a love for animals". Well if I didn't want the job before that I sure did after. I accepted the job with a welcoming handshake and was sorry but I had to work my notice first. I knew this was going to be the beginning of a fantastic job and friendship, I couldn't wait to start.

Andrea was upset because I was leaving, as was little Jane I assured them we would still be friends, but I knew as they did that we would soon drift apart. In a funny sort of way I would miss the co-op, for it really opened my world, but as I knew from the very first day it was not the job for me.

I had since Prince and Mindy found a deep love for animals, I cared very much for even the smallest ones, I had taken many injured ones home for dad and me to save, not that many did but it wasn't for lack of trying. Mindy taught me that animals don't judge they love you if you're well or ill, they sense your need for love, and like Mindy they repay it ten fold. Over the many years of pleasure my Mindy bought me, even at my most ill I was never mean or nasty to her, she was always my friend.

The night before I was to start my new life. I went to "my Lindsay". I felt a bit guilty, for I did not visit her as much as I should do. But she didn't seem to mind; she was just really pleased I was so happy. I felt so very different now that I was an

adult. For Lindsay was like a little kid sister, but she is myself at the age I put her into her safe room. She can never grow old, get ill, die she is everything that was pure to me innocent without evil, not like an angel she is nothing like that just a perfect innocent child. My Lindsay has been my friend since I can remember and it's nice to know that even though I am an adult, I can still go to her for my inner peace. To know that we will be together until we die is very satisfying.

I bought myself a second hand pushbike from the bike shop on Friday, so on Monday morning in my overall and wellies I could ride to my new job to begin another chapter in my life.

Chapter Thirteen

I just can't begin to tell you just how wonderful Meadow Brooke Farm is, the birds are the most wonderful creatures I have ever seen; their colours, shapes, and elegance and grace give such an air about them. I stand watching them with such joy in my heart. To be honest I was never interested in birds of any sort but now all I want to do is to learn as much as I can about each of the different species. Mrs Hall or Mrs H as I call her is a very nice employer. She teaches me things about the birds that you couldn't find in books, she also gives me time just to watch them, how many there are I could only hazard a guess, about five hundred plus, maybe more some are more rarer than others, but all get treated the same. It takes me about an hour and half morning and evening to feed and check all the birds. The six foot high fence enclosures with the three manmade ponds in them, covers about two and a half acres. Mrs H told me that they started of with one pond, and that it took three days for the digger to dig the hole. All three large ponds run into one another, around them and in between them are banks, plants, reeds and trees and they have all been planted by Mrs H and the farm workers. The whole massive enclosure, birds and all are the most interesting and beautiful place anyone could wish to be; I feel so honoured to be working here.

The sheep are very boring, I take water to them in big plastic drums each day, and walk

among them making sure they are all fit and healthy, (not that in my early days I knew what I was looking for). Mrs H told me that tupping and lambing was the most interesting time of year for the sheep. I suppose that the fact that they run away from you, even though I was friend not foe, didn't help a new comer to find them interesting, as time went on I felt they would grow on me.

The real hold on me was the pleasure I had felt being with all the birds, and Mrs H, she had become a person I had a lot of respect for.

The first six months Mrs H asked a lot of questions about why I had left the pig farm. About dad (being my foster dad) I was caught off guard once, and nearly realised my sordid past, but somehow I always managed to fob her off, after six months or so she stopped asking. I wanted to be just a normal person and I knew that if Mrs H found out about my past, that she wouldn't give me the respect that I knew I could earn from her in time.

Mother was very quiet, I think it is because she is getting old and her powers over me were becoming weaker. But I suppose dad could have something in these pills, he was making me take, who cares I was having a break I didn't want to know WHY, I was just so grateful for the peace. If I wasn't at work then I had my nose in books that I had bought, I found that with dad helping me, I could learn a great deal about each of the different

breeds of birds that I spent my days with. I learnt about all the different sizes, weights and colours of their eggs, for the more I learnt the more I wanted to learn. A duck to me had the best life of any animal. The skill of swimming and diving and the freedom to take to the air and go wherever it wanted, dad understood my new passion for my feathered friends we were so alike dad and me, almost like real father and daughter.

My dad was always up before I left for work, but not this morning instead ma got me my coffee, she said "dad was having a lay in" and off I went to work quite happily. Not one thought had crossed my mind that maybe my dad was "not well". Even when Mrs H sent for me in the middle of feeding, I still never thought anything was wrong. When she took my hand and told me that my dad was being rushed to hospital and that she would drive me, it was so unreal my mind just went blank. I felt from Mrs H something was very wrong, but I didn't let myself believe it. We arrived just as the ambulance with dad and ma in it pulled up as my dad was taken out by stretcher, ma thanked Mrs H for bringing me. Within fifteen minutes we were told dad was in a coma. We were taken to a side room of one of the male wards and we had to wait ages till we could see him and was warned about machines, drips and tubes but that didn't prepare us for what he was like. Ma and me sat at each side of his bed both of us touching his hands, tears was streaming down our faces, just kept on thinking my dads alright,

he's just asleep. For the rest of the day we sat in silence for we needed no words, both of us praying in our own way that this man who we both loved so dearly would wake up and want to know what all the fuss was about. Nurses and doctors came and left, after one doctor-examined dad he asked if he could talk to ma outside.

While ma was outside talking dad's eyes suddenly opened and called for ma and I gently stroked my dad's face. He was trying to say something and leaned forward to hear his words, just as ma came bursting back into the room dad said three words to me before his eyes closed **"look after ma"**. Nurses came in and checked dad. Ma and I stood in the corner of his room. Watching them seeing to dad. I told ma in a whisper what dad had said and automatically regretted it, for her face if possible showed more sorrow than she already had. We sat with dad all evening just praying that he would wake up again, but at ten to midnight the night nurse came in and after checking all the machines and tubes, turned to ma and me and said "we should go home and get some sleep". I started to say "no way" then she carried on and said "he was sleeping peacefully and if there was any change at all she would ring us straight away". We looked at each other we were both indeed shattered, and Mindy had been shut in for over eighteen hours. We both decided the nurse was right, so after a long good bye we told dad we would see him in the morning. When I kissed him he felt so nice and warm, we

made sure they had the right number and we left the ward to return home.

The taxi man would not shut up, although it was only a short journey, I just wanted to yell at him that my dad was really ill, and that the last thing we both needed was all his questions. But I didn't, for the last thing ma would want was a scene. Mindy had messed in the kitchen by the back door, I cleaned it up and then I fed her, while ma made sandwiches and a hot drink. We were both deep in our own thoughts to say very much at all. Neither of us could eat anything, but our drinks were very welcoming. Mindy laid by my feet, she knew there was something very wrong, ma suggested that we both slept in the front room, to be nearer to the phone (we only had one telephone and it was in the downstairs hall). Ma got some covers and without getting undressed we laid down to rest, praying dad was still comfortable. As I lay there I never once thought that my dad would not be alright, death was not even a glancing thought. I had never thought about life without my dad and ma.

I must have slept for I awoke to the sound of the phone ringing. Ma got to it first and I could hear a female voice on the other end talking. Ma "**cried out**" and fell back onto the bottom stair with the phone still in her hand; her face was one of total shock and disbelief I started shouting at her to tell me, but she remained silent. I heard a voice from the phone and snatched it from her, I was

shouting down it for them to tell me what's wrong, the voice said "calm down then we can talk, take deep breaths" is your mum with you the nurse asked yes I said she's just staring at me, please, please tell me is my dad alright? She told me "that my dad had passed away peacefully in his sleep". My body slid down the wall and the phone fell somewhere on the floor, I like ma had no words to say. The tears came later as ma sat on the floor and cuddled me we cried and sobbed together for the loss of the most wonderful man who had ever walked this earth. I even told ma, that I hated him for leaving us. Ma made a drink and we sat together on the settee, both in the state of shock, it was over four hours later that ma phoned her sister to tell her of dads death, Still in yesterdays clothes we sat in our front room with two of Ma's sisters and her brother all of them, wanting to know, Why and How, Ma told them what had happened and in disbelief they sat and shared in our sorrow he was my dad for only seven short years, but in that time he had given me a life time full of love. He was and still is the most wonderful man God ever made, for he did not only love me he taught me, he moulded me into the person who would someday make him proud. But what for "he's dead" he's left me, he's abandoned me, what was all the fighting for, what was life for. Sometimes I hated him for leaving me alone in this horrible world, but I soon realised that he had given me a job to do, like a quest really **"look after ma, look after ma"** they were his last words to me, and because of the love for him I knew I

would honour them. The following week was **hell** arranging the funeral, picking hymns, arranging flowers; dad didn't like wasting money on things that just died, so we had family flowers only, donations to the save the children fund. We both knew he would be happy with that. During the first week I felt maybe at times, that ma blamed me why I didn't know. On the fourth day I just came out and asked her, she cuddled me so tight I had trouble getting my breath, she said the time I was his daughter was his happiest, that I had fulfilled a dream, and that he felt because he had passed so much of himself onto me that his life had been given a purpose. I hugged ma feeling my fears had not been needed.

The day of the funeral was indeed the worst day of ma's and my life until that day I felt it all could be a mistake, but it is very final when the coffin goes down behind those curtains, I felt sick to my stomach ma cried the whole day, I did (but more inside than out). Because dad's words were etched in my brain. Most of the people that day I didn't know, but each and every one of them knew and loved the man I am so proud to call **my dad**.

And there my story must end. To live without the one true person I loved and who understood me, would be impossibility.

Dad made me who I am without him nothing matters; death was not something except for my friend that I had encountered before.

My life, my world has become so empty, meaningless and yet I some how know I will have to go on. Dads final words to me would make sure I did, I often wonder did he know that he was dying, if so did he say these words to keep me alive for he was indeed a man with great insight.

The first half of my life stops here, my journey into adulthood begins in my next book; it's a journey so full of nightmares of my child hood and my mental illness.

Will I ever have a life without mother? Can I ever be normal, do normal things like get married, have a family or will I rot in a hospital ward somewhere tormented forever, by a mother so evil that her only true wish is to see her daughter suffer?

Writing this book has been the hardest thing I have ever done. But I pray that by doing so, I can help in some small way to give insight into what child abuse can lead to. Most adults with a mental illness have suffered child abuse as children. Also to the staff, nurses and doctors to read the other side of the coin maybe helpful.
Thank you.

www.ingramcontent.com/pod-product-compliance
Lightning Source LLC
Chambersburg PA
CBHW022127080426
42734CB00006B/256